Health Financing in Ghana

Health Financing in Ghana

George Schieber, Cheryl Cashin, Karima Saleh, and Rouselle Lavado

THE WORLD BANK
Washington, D.C.

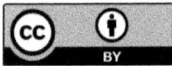

Contents

Box

Figures

Tables

Foreword

Ghana is one of a small number of African countries that has passed legislation, earmarked significant revenues, and seriously begun implementation of a public health insurance program for its entire population. The national program, which was scaled up from smaller community-based health insurance schemes, has tried to include poor and vulnerable population groups in the first stages of implementation by exempting these groups from contributions and providing earmarked financing for their coverage. However, Ghana has faced considerable challenges along the way.

Developing the institutions and policies that can successfully support complex national mandatory health insurance programs has not been easy, even for high-income countries with robust institutions and technical know-how. For emerging market countries, the challenges are formidable—designing an affordable basic benefits package; targeting vulnerable groups; developing health management information systems for enrollment, claims processing, and payment; implementing results-based provider payment mechanisms; guaranteeing quality and controlling fraud and abuse; assuring the availability of needed health services; and ensuring the long-term financial sustainability of the scheme.

In seven years, Ghana has made substantial progress in terms of institutional development, implementation of the insurance program, and improving access to essential health services. However, with many Ghanaians still lacking coverage, costs outrunning contributions, and the threat of financial insolvency in the years ahead, Ghanaian health policymakers are now at a crossroads.

This comprehensive study is designed to assist Ghana by suggesting a number of options to reform the structural and operational features of Ghana's National Health Insurance Scheme to ensure its smooth transition to universal coverage and financial sustainability. Policy options are based on an analytical assessment of how Ghana's health system is performing—whether it meets basic goals such as improving health outcomes, financial protection, consumer responsiveness, equity, efficiency, and sustainability. Health financing reform options are developed in the context of Ghana's health system configuration as well as its demographic, epidemiological, socioeconomic, labor-market, industrial-structure, political, and geographic realities.

This is a critical moment for Ghana's efforts to get health care to all Ghanaians. Actions taken in the next two years will determine if this effort succeeds. It is hoped that this study will contribute to Ghana's success.

Ritva S. Reinikka, Sector Director
Human Development, Africa Region
World Bank

Acknowledgments

The report was prepared by a team led by Karima Saleh. The principal authors are George Schieber, Cheryl Cashin, Karima Saleh, and Rouselle Lavado. Contributions were received from Angela Micah, Moulay Driss Zine Eddine El Idrissi, Francois Diop, Ronald Hendriks, Andreas Seiter, Iryna Postolovska, and Dennis Streveler.

The team appreciates the comments from peer reviewers John Langenbrunner, Maureen Lewis, Gayle Martin, Somil Nagpal, and Netsanet Walelign. The team also received comments from Sebastien Dessus and Felix Oppong. The team is grateful for the valuable input of the Health Financing Technical Sub-Committee for the Ghana Country Status Report[1] and the many other government officials, development partners, and private sector professionals who contributed their time, data, and insights. The team would also like to thank the participants in a series of workshops held in Accra in June 2011 and January 2012 for their valuable comments and suggestions. Special thanks go to Mr. Sylvester A. Mensah, Chief Executive of the National Health Insurance Authority (NHIA), and his staff for their insightful feedback on the initial draft report, which was presented at a special

NHIA workshop in June 2011. The team would also like to thank the leadership and staffs of the Ministry of Health, the Ghana Health Service, the Ministry of Finance and Economic Planning, and the Parliamentary Select Committee on Health for their valuable comments on the draft report.

---

[1] Karima Saleh, *The Health Sector in Ghana: A Comprehensive Assessment* (Washington, DC: World Bank, forthcoming [2012]).

About the Authors

George Schieber is a public finance economist with a Ph.D. in economics and more than 30 years of experience in over 60 countries. Prior to his current work as an independent consultant, he served as sector manager for health and social protection for the World Bank's Middle East and North Africa Region, director of the Office of Research and Demonstrations of the U.S. Health Care Financing Administration, administrator at the Organisation for Economic Co-operation and Development (OECD), research economist at the Urban Institute, and assistant professor of economics at the University of Pittsburgh. He has written over 60 books and articles including the World Bank's *Health Financing Revisited* (2006) and *Good Practices in Health Financing* (2008).

Cheryl Cashin is a health economist with more than 20 years of experience working on health financing policy design, implementation and evaluation in low- and middle-income countries. She holds a Ph.D. in economics from the University of Washington and an M.S. from Cornell University. She is currently a senior fellow at Results for Development Institute, leading the Provider Payment Technical Track of the Joint Learning Network for Universal Health Coverage. She is a coauthor of the World Bank's publications *Designing and Implementing Health Care Provider Payment Systems: How-to Manuals* (2009) and "Assessing Public Expenditure on Health from a Fiscal Space Perspective" (2010).

Karima Saleh is a health economist with over 15 years of experience in over 15 countries. She holds a Ph.D. in health economics from the Johns Hopkins University. She is currently a senior economist (health) at the World Bank, with work experience (including field work) on health financing policy in low- and low-middle income countries. She was part of the core team that developed the 1993 World Development Report, *Investing in Health*, and has several publications forthcoming in the World Bank's Directions in Development series, including *The Health Sector in Ghana: A Comprehensive Assessment.*

Rouselle Lavado is a senior fellow at the Institute for Health Metrics and Evaluation (IHME) and senior research fellow at the Philippine Institute for Development Studies. At IHME, she is part of the Health Financing Research team, developing methods to estimate private expenditure on health. She has also worked at the Asian Development Bank Institute and the Policy Center of the Asian Institute of Management and as a consultant for the World Bank, the World Health Organization, the German Agency for Technical Cooperation (GTZ), and the United States Agency for International Development. She received her master's and doctorate degrees in public policy at Hitotsubashi University, Japan.

Abbreviations

CHPS	community-based health program and services
CSR	Country Status Report
DALY	disability adjusted life year
DMHIS	district mutual health insurance scheme
GDP	gross domestic product
G-DRG	Ghana Diagnosis Related Group
GHS	Ghana Health Service
GLSS	Ghana Living Standards Survey
HMIS	health management information system
MDG	Millennium Development Goal
MOFEP	Ministry of Finance and Economic Planning
NHA	National Health Accounts
NHIA	National Health Insurance Authority
NHIF	National Health Insurance Fund
NHIL	National Health Insurance Levy
NHIS	National Health Insurance Scheme
OECD	Organisation for Economic Co-operation and Development
SSNIT	Social Security and National Insurance Trust
VAT	value added tax

Overview

This report reviews Ghana's health financing system, with a special emphasis on its National Health Insurance Scheme (NHIS). The study also undertakes for the first time an extensive international benchmarking analysis, assesses the financial protection/equity of the system at both the macro and micro levels, and analyzes Ghana's fiscal space in the wake of its reclassification as a lower-middle-income country in November 2010.

The report is particularly important because Ghana is often considered an example of global "good practice," as it is one of only a handful of emerging market countries in Africa to actively start implementing universal health insurance coverage by providing formal coverage to its vulnerable population groups. The report is also timely, in view of a recent critique of the NHIS (and a call to abandon it in favor of a national health service) as well as the publication of several new and updated sources of information on total health spending, inputs, outcomes, household spending, and the macroeconomy.

Study Approach

The report addresses five key areas:

- It describes demographic and epidemiological trends in Ghana; the configuration of Ghana's health system, the functions of health financing, and the goals of health systems; and Ghana's health financing system.
- It assesses the performance of Ghana's health system by comparing its health outcomes, inputs, health spending, and financial protection with comparator countries.
- Based on this assessment and the significant body of Ghana-specific health policy literature, it analyzes the strengths and weaknesses of Ghana's health system, providing a baseline for reform.
- It assesses the sustainability of the NHIS in the context of Ghana's future fiscal space, based on revised macroeconomic information positioning Ghana as a lower-middle-income country.
- It identifies major structural and operational reform options for ensuring the long-term efficacy and sustainability of the NHIS.

Key Messages

The report yields four key messages:

1. Ghana's health financing system is going in the right direction based on international good practices. There is a clear movement away from supply-side subsidies toward demand-side financing, the revenue sources of the NHIS are diversified and progressive, and substantial resources are allocated to ensure coverage of vulnerable groups. The NHIS appears to have reduced financial access barriers to health care, increased utilization, and been pro-poor, although some equity issues remain. It is functioning as a new unified health purchaser with a maturing strategic purchasing function that, although not yet adequately exploited, has the potential to be a force for change and modernization in service delivery.

2. As a share of GDP, total health spending in Ghana is slightly below average for a lower-middle-income country; public spending is about average. Despite this spending, the under-five mortality rate and maternal mortality ratio are higher than in comparator countries.

3. Modest increases in government expenditure on health will be possible as a result of economic growth and improved revenue collection measures.

As a result of the earmarked National Health Insurance Levy (NHIL) and social security contributions, the health sector (and the NHIS in particular) will likely get at least its share of any new revenues, and slightly more as Ghana evolves to a middle-income country and expands its share of GDP allocated to health.

4. The system has serious structural and operational inefficiencies and is on a trajectory to go bankrupt as early as 2013. For the NHIS to expand enrollment and become sustainable, more public resources will be needed. The system is too inefficient to absorb significant new resources, however; without major reforms, some of which lie outside the purview of the NHIS, it is difficult to argue for major increases in funding, particularly given Ghana's fragile macroeonomic/fiscal situation. Fundamental reforms are needed to coverage rules, the basic benefit package, provider payment, and cost control to ensure efficient use of resources and bring expenditures into closer alignment with available resources and Ghana's future fiscal space.

Health System Performance

Population growth and structural changes will strongly affect Ghana's health financing needs as well as its ability to meet those needs. Ghana's population will increase by almost 40 percent by 2030—but the number of people 65 and older will increase by 90 percent. The burden of disease will continue to shift from communicable diseases to noncommunicable diseases and injuries. In the medium term, Ghana will have to deal with the dual burden of disease, which will impose significant costs on the health system. The fact that an estimated 70–90 percent of Ghana's labor force works in the informal sector and that most firms are very small provides significant challenges to both revenue collection and enrollment in the NHIS.

The performance of Ghana's health system is mixed. Consumer satisfaction is high, and access appears to have improved, including for the poor. Total health spending as a share of GDP is slightly below the global average for countries at the comparable level of income, however; Ghana has fewer hospital beds and health workers and worse under-five and maternal mortality outcomes than comparator countries; and health spending increased less rapidly than spending in most African counties between 1995 and 2009. Since 2004, public health spending increased 11 percent faster than GDP and 15 percent faster than government revenues. Despite these increases, the share of the government budget dedicated to health is below the 15 percent Abuja target, as it is in many other African countries.

Specific findings from the performance assessment include the following:

- For countries at its level of income and health spending, Ghana performs worse than average with respect to under-five (and infant) mortality and maternal mortality but better than average for life expectancy.
- Over the past several decades, improvements in some health outcomes in Ghana have been less impressive than in several neighboring countries, despite starting from better levels.
- Ghana has fewer physicians and health workers per capita than other countries with comparable income and health spending. It also has a serious shortage of specialists.
- In 2009, Ghana had fewer hospital beds per capita than other countries with comparable income and health spending.
- Over the past several decades, increases in hospital beds and physicians per capita have been smaller than in many neighboring countries; since 1985, the increase in the number of hospital beds has not kept pace with population growth in Ghana.
- Ghana spends less than 5 percent of its GDP on health, slightly below average for a country at its income level.
- According to the 2009 World Health Organization (WHO) National Health Accounts, 47 percent of total health spending in Ghana is private (37 percent paid out of pocket and 10 percent paid by private insurance and other private risk-pooling mechanisms).
- Of the 53 percent public spending share, the NHIS accounts for some 30 percent of public spending on health and 16 percent of total health spending.
- Depending on how it is measured, public spending on health in Ghana is either slightly above or about the same as global income comparators.
- Depending on how it is measured, out-of-pocket spending (a gross measure of financial protection) in Ghana is higher than or about the same as global income comparators but twice the threshold recommended by the WHO.
- From an equity perspective, enrollment in the NHIS appears to have led to better utilization by the poor of health facilities, and financing appears to be progressive. The incidence of enrollment and overall benefits do not appear to be pro-poor, however.

Health System Strengths and Weakness

Ghana's health system has important strengths but also faces major challenges. Strengths include the following.

Governance, management, and organization

- The government has in place the administrative and legal requirements
  for its decentralized governance structure.
- The public financial management system is adequate and clear, and it
  meets most international requirements.
- Successive common management arrangements provide an effective
  framework for relating to partners.
- The NHIS legislation (Act 650) strategically sets out an elaborate governance and administrative framework for the provision of health
  insurance.
- Consumer satisfaction with the NHIS is high.

Delivery system, pharmaceuticals, and public health

- There have been large increases in human resources for health and
  production of nurses, and the production of doctors is higher than
  many countries in the region.
- Exits from the labor market have been largely the result of retirement,
  not outmigration, since the 2006 salary increase.
- Informal payments are reportedly uncommon, although anecdotal evidence and the high out-of-pocket share of total health spending suggest
  the need for in-depth analysis of this issue.
- The Ministry of Health and the Ghana Health Service have developed
  a comprehensive approach to set priorities for investments, considering
  recurrent costs, human resource constraints, maintenance implications,
  and other factors.
- Utilization of outpatient departments has increased significantly.
- Hospital use trends for most categories are positive, with occupancy
  rates increasing from 45 percent to 60 percent and average lengths of
  stay decreasing from 4.5 to 3.8 days between 2005 and 2009.
- A vibrant private sector is a major supplier of all forms of nonhospital
  care and a significant supplier of hospital care.
- Ghana has a reasonable essential drugs list and good availability of
  drugs.

- Full immunization coverage has increased, HIV/AIDS prevalence is low, and Ghana is likely to meet the Millenium Development Goals (MDG) target for child nutrition.

Financing

- Ghana is one of very few emerging market countries to take serious steps toward demand-side financing for health, pass legislation for universal health insurance coverage, begin implementation by covering vulnerable groups, significantly expand enrollment, and earmark substantial resources to support the system.
- The revenue base for Ghana's overall health financing system is largely progressive, and the NHIS relies on a diversified set of largely progressive funding sources, resulting in significant and stable sources of revenues.
- Ghana's approach is pragmatically built on its existing system of community-based health insurance plans transitioned into district mutual health insurance schemes (DMHISs) and is evolving toward a uniform national system.
- According to the NHIS, active membership in 2010 was 8.16 million, some 34 percent of the population. Since 2005, outpatient visits have increased by a factor of 23, inpatient service by a factor of 29, and expenditures by a factor of 40.

Ghana's health system also includes a variety of weaknesses. These weaknesses include the following.

Governance, management, and organization

- The decentralized health sector faces a number of serious challenges, including potential inconsistencies between the government's overall model of devolution versus the Ghana Health Service's model of deconcentration.
- Local authorities have little control over budgets/expenditures, because most of their resources are executed centrally or earmarked from the center to specific programs or initiatives.
- Health workforce ratios are low; health infrastructure, equipment, transport, and the health management information system (HMIS) are inadequate; drug procurement is inefficient and the performance of the central medical stores is poor; and financing, quality assurance, and logistics management are weak.

- Weak coordination by the various regulatory agencies results in high drug prices and substandard drugs.

Delivery system, pharmaceuticals, and public health

- Health care provider densities are far below the levels recommended by the WHO.
- The number of health care workers is inadequate, and staff, especially high-level cadres, are underrepresented in rural areas and areas with high poverty levels.
- Few incentives are in place to ensure the performance of health sector workers.
- Hospital occupancy rates have increased to 60 percent, but there is considerable interregional variation in occupancy rates, the number of beds, average lengths of stay, and turnover, suggesting less than optimal allocation and use of this expensive input.
- Expansion of health infrastructure is limited by inadequate financial resources; delays in the release of budgetary allocations, resulting in cost overruns; unplanned initiation of projects outside the capital investment plan; weak planned preventive maintenance; and problems with the acquisition, distribution, installation, and use of equipment.
- District health and subdistrict health systems are weak and lack a focus on primary care.
- Ghana is unlikely to meet the MDG target for maternal mortality; anemia is a major problem among women and children; the contraceptive prevalence rate is low and stagnant, with high levels of unmet needs, and the prevalence of tuberculosis is high and stagnant, with large unmet needs.

Financing

- Given its current expenditure and expansion plans, the NHIS is not financially viable and is projected to be insolvent possibly as early as 2013.
- Premiums, taxes, and reinsurance payments for the NHIS and to the DMHISs are not actuarially determined, and premiums for informal sector workers are low relative to their costs.
- The original health insurance law does not require a reserve fund, which is critical to a program like the NHIS.

- The basic benefit package is heavily biased toward curative care, coordination with Ministry of Health vertical programs is poor, and coverage of 95 percent of the burden of disease with no cost sharing may not be affordable.
- Lack of an effective gatekeeper system, an ineffective referral system, and misaligned provider payment incentives prevent the NHIS from being an effective "active" purchaser.
- A significant proportion (perhaps on the order of 30 percent) of the 65 percent of people who are exempt from paying premiums could afford to contribute.
- The stringent definition of indigent excludes some poor and near-poor.
- Lack of a modern HMIS results in poor claims management and quality assurance, high administrative costs, and incomplete information on enrollees and providers.

Fiscal Space

Options for health reform in Ghana are constrained by the country's future available fiscal space. An extensive assessment of fiscal space undertaken as part of this study indicates that economic growth and improved revenue collection efforts could provide modest but steady increases in fiscal space for health over the next three to five years. New fiscal space will be possible, however, only if Ghana achieves a collection rate of 20 percent of GDP by 2015.

Adding significant new expenditure burdens to the fragile macroeconomic and fiscal recovery is not realistic. Furthermore, prudent public policy indicates that countries should not raise additional revenues to increase spending in a system that is inefficient. Thus, increases in resources for the NHIS are likely to have to come from within the system, through efficiency gains from more rational expenditure patterns.

Reform Options

Based on the analyses of performance and fiscal space, this report suggests several potential options for reform:

1. At least maintain the share allocated to the health sector of any new revenue, either from economic growth or improved revenue collection.

2. Ensure that the full amount of commitments from all sources is transferred to the NHIS in a timely manner.
3. Optimize the mobilization of resources within the NHIS through enforced means-tested premiums and possibly strategic copayments to both add to the revenue base and direct utilization toward more cost-effective services.
4. Revisit the NHIS eligibility and benefit package to be sure they are rational given economic realities in Ghana. The comprehensive benefit package may be sustainable if it is combined with appropriate cost sharing and serious provider payment/cost containment reforms.
5. Embark on an effective strategy of purchasing within the NHIS to use provider payment systems and other purchasing tools to contain cost growth, improve the cost-effectiveness of service utilization, and drive greater efficiencies in the health system.
6. Address the severe operational inefficiencies within the NHIS, particularly claims-processing bottlenecks and the slow process of automation and HMIS modernization.
7. Address inefficiencies in the health service delivery system, particularly high administrative costs and low productivity of health workers.
8. Examine the large transfer of funds from the NHIS budget to the Ministry of Health. It is not clear why such large transfers are necessary or whether the funds could be more effectively used to augment demand-side financing and cover a larger share of the health system's operating costs through the provider payment mechanisms of the NHIS.

The report argues that replacing the NHIS with a national health service would not fix the system's problems. It shows that the fundamental design features and operational policies of the NHIS share many of the advantages often attributed to a national health service (for example, progressive general revenue funding, coverage of vulnerable groups) and that current policy directions will endow the NHIS with the basic advantages of a formal health insurance model in terms of strategic purchasing and purchaser-provider splits. Refining the structural and operational features of the NHIS to ensure its evolution as an effective public insurance organization is a much more sensible approach than going back to a fully general revenue–funded national health service with free care to all provided through a publically owned and operated delivery system.

Table O.1   Options for Reforming Ghana's National Health Insurance Scheme

Issue	*Option*
Eligibility for premium subsidies and enrollment changes	• Focus on the poor • Change the eligibility unit from the individual to the household • Create incentives to encourage enrollment
Basic benefits package	• Review extensiveness • Consider cost sharing for the nonpoor • Coordinate with vertical public health programs
Revenues	• Increase the VAT earmark • Increase the SSNIT contribution • Impose sin taxes • Means test exempt groups • Levy a one-time premium on enrollees
Provider payment	• Implement payment systems that encourage efficiency, quality, cost-effective service utilization, and better coordination across the continuum of care; options include the appropriate mix of capitation, other bundled payment systems, blended payment systems, various managed care approaches, and modern pay-for-performance systems
Pharmaceuticals	• Establish more rational reimbursement methods, including capitation for basic primary care medicines, bundling by G-DRGs, reference pricing, or other modern reimbursement methods • Improve information systems and introduce incentives for the rational use of medicines • Update the drug list, based on medical appropriateness criteria • Reduce expenditure for generic medicines through pooled procurement • Consider appropriate copayments • Provide consumer and provider education
Administrative reforms	• Provide data for decision making • Improve the HMIS • Centralize control • Adopt other operational reforms
Other	• Strengthen public health • Invest in physical and human infrastructure • Improve governance

Source: Authors.

The report analyzes specific policy options for increasing revenues and improving expenditure efficiency in the context of broader reforms of the health systems. Table O.1 summarizes possible reforms.

The NHIS is at a crossroads. The government needs to act decisively to ensure the sustainability and efficacy of the system. In a short time,

Ghana has made substantial progress in transitioning the NHIS into a functioning health insurance program for a significant part of its population. Its future now depends on strategic health policy choices and an effective transition to universal coverage. These choices will determine whether the NHIS becomes an effective health insurance entity for the entire Ghanaian population and an example of global best practice or just another stage in Ghana's quest for universal coverage.

CHAPTER 1

Introduction

This report reviews Ghana's health financing system, with a special emphasis on its National Health Insurance Scheme (NHIS).[1] It focuses on broad structural financing issues. The report is an input into *The Health Sector in Ghana: A Comprehensive Assessment* (Saleh forthcoming [2012]) (also referred to as the 2012 Ghana Country Status Report [CSR]) and the government's ongoing health financing reform efforts. As health financing interacts with all other health systems components, this report also relies on other CSR background reports as well as on the prodigious literature on Ghana.

The intent of this report is not to replicate other efforts but to provide an up-to-date assessment of Ghana's health financing system given the rapid expansion of the NHIS since its legislative inception in 2003–04 and its implementation in 2005. Ghana's innovative approach to universal coverage is also being closely watched globally, as it is one of the few African countries to begin implementation by covering its vulnerable populations, earmarking significant national revenues to finance the system, and moving to a uniform national system by scaling up and integrating its district mutual health insurance schemes.

This report is timely, as several new sources of data have become available, including information on total health spending, inputs, outcomes, household spending, and the macroeconomy (the significant macroeconomic revisions of November 2010, which resulted in Ghana's reclassification as a lower-middle-income country). It undertakes for the first time an extensive international benchmarking analysis, in which health outcomes, inputs, and financing system features in Ghana are compared with other countries with similar levels of income or spending on health care; assesses changes over time in the financial protection/equity of the system at both the macro and micro levels; and provides an extensive analysis of fiscal space based on Ghana's new macroeconomic realities.

The report is divided into five chapters. This chapter provides background on demographic and epidemiological trends, the configuration of Ghana's health system, and health financing functions and health systems goals. It also describes Ghana's health financing system. Chapter 2 assesses the performance of Ghana's health system with respect to these goals through international comparisons of health outcomes, inputs, spending, and financial protection as well as time series comparisons of trends in other countries in Africa. Chapter 3 identifies the strengths and weaknesses of Ghana's health system, which determine Ghana's health reform baseline. Chapter 4 analyzes the sustainability of the NHIS in the context of Ghana's future fiscal space, based on Ghana's new standing as a lower-middle-income country. Chapter 5 analyzes major structural and operational reform options that will help ensure the long-term efficacy and sustainability of the NHIS.

Underlying Demographics and Epidemiology

Ghana's underlying demographics and epidemiological situations are important determinants not only of the health system's future needs/demands but also of the ability of its population to support those needs/demands (for example, the ratio of people of working age to the elderly and young). Figure 1.1 shows the population pyramids for Ghana in 2010 and 2030.

Ghana's population will increase from its 2010 level of 24.3 million to 33.8 million in 2030, an increase of 39 percent. With declining birth rates and increasing life expectancy, the percentage of the population below 14 will decrease from 38.1 percent in 2010 to 30.8 percent in 2030, and the percentage of the population over 64 will increase from 3.7 percent to 5.0 percent. In 2030, there will be 90 percent more people over 64 in Ghana than there were in 2010 (World Bank HNP STATS, accessed April 21, 2011). Ghana's health system and other social programs will need to grow to meet the increasing demands of the country's growing and structurally changing population.

Figure 1.1   Ghana Population Pyramids, 2010 and 2030

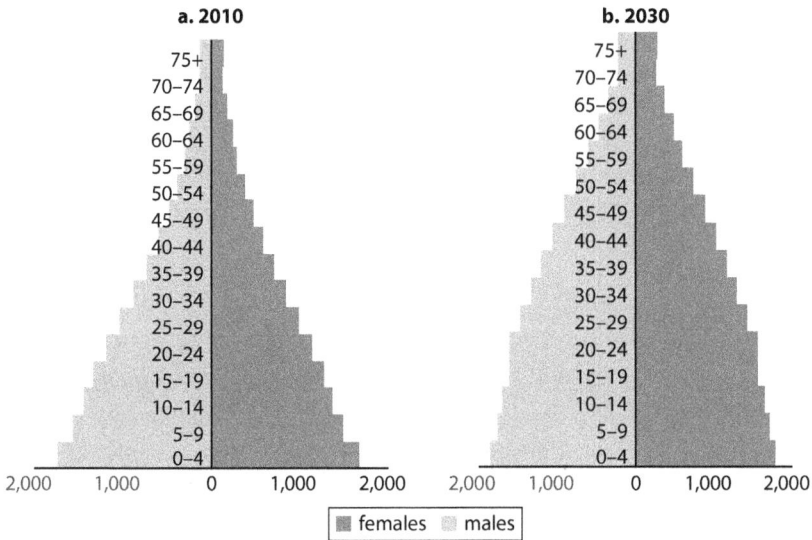

a. 2010

b. 2030

females   males

Source: World Bank HNP STATS, accessed April 24, 2011.

Another important aspect of this changing population structure relates to "population momentum." As a result of Ghana's past high rates of population growth, large numbers of people will be entering the "productive" labor force age range of 14–64, fewer babies will be born, and more people will be entering the 64-plus age range. The number of dependents per person of productive age will decline from 0.72 in 2010 to 0.56 in 2030 and 0.51 in 2050. The "demographic dividend" from this falling dependency ratio will be reaped only if Ghana can productively employ these people.

Future employment, productivity growth, and revenue will also depend on the size distribution of firms as well as the level of informality in the economy. Currently, 70 percent of firms in Ghana have fewer than five employees, and 70–90 percent of the labor force may be in the informal sector (Ghana Statistical Service and WIEGO 2005; Benzing and Hung 2009). These factors are partially responsible for Ghana's current (and possible future) low revenues and premium collection. If Ghana cannot productively employ people entering the labor force, the demographic dividend could turn into a demographic curse, leading to lower growth, tax revenues, and NHIS premium income, as well as political unrest.

As a result of the demographic transition, the pattern and burden of disease in Ghana will change (the "epidemiological transition"). Assuming it follows the Sub-Saharan African trend, Ghana's burden of disease will continue shifting from communicable to noncommunicable diseases and injuries over the next 20 years (figure 1.2). The communicable disease burden is projected to decline from 52 percent to 39 percent, while the noncommunicable disease burden is projected to increase from 41 percent to 47 percent. The burden of injuries and accidents is projected to increase from 7 percent to 14 percent.

Noncommunicable diseases and injuries are much more expensive to treat and require different health system inputs. In the absence of effective road and occupational safety, disease prevention, and health promotion strategies, as well as much better coordination between the Ministry of Health/Ghana Health Service and the NHIS, the epidemiological transition will exacerbate impending cost pressures on, necessitate major modifications to, and significantly increase the financing needs of Ghana's health system. The little-discussed nutrition transition (malnutrition as a continuing serious problem along with increasing overnutrition) will exacerbate Ghana's future noncommunicable disease burden. Although not the focus of this report, these are important areas for Ghana's health reform agenda.

Configuration of Ghana's Health System

Ghana has a well-developed, integrated, multilevel health system distributed throughout the country. The system comprises community-based

Figure 1.2   Burden of Disease in Ghana (Actual) and Sub-Saharan Africa (Projected)

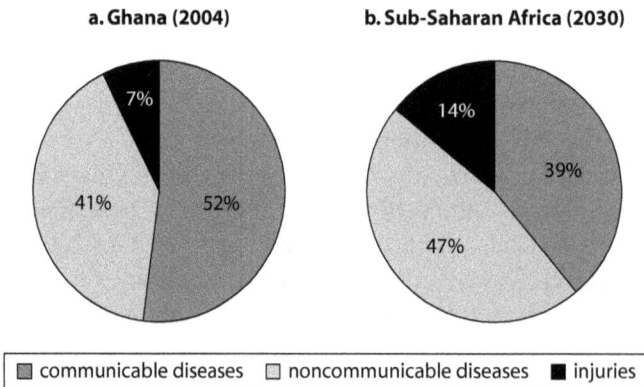

a. Ghana (2004)   b. Sub-Saharan Africa (2030)

■ communicable diseases   □ noncommunicable diseases   ■ injuries

Source: WHO 2008.

health planning and services zones; health centers; district, regional, and teaching hospitals; private health providers; and nongovernmental health-related organizations (figure 1.3). The Ministry of Health is the steward of the system, which consists of public (the Ghana Health Service), nongovernmental organization (the Christian Health Association of Ghana [CHAG]), and private providers, as well as the National Health Insurance Authority (NHIA) and numerous governmental and regulatory entities at various levels of Ghana's highly decentralized health system (figure 1.4).

Human resources for health have increased significantly in Ghana, where the production of nurses and doctors is higher than in many countries in the region (Appiah and others forthcoming). Ghana has a vibrant private sector that supplies all forms of nonhospital care and a significant share

Figure 1.3   Organization of Ghana's Health System

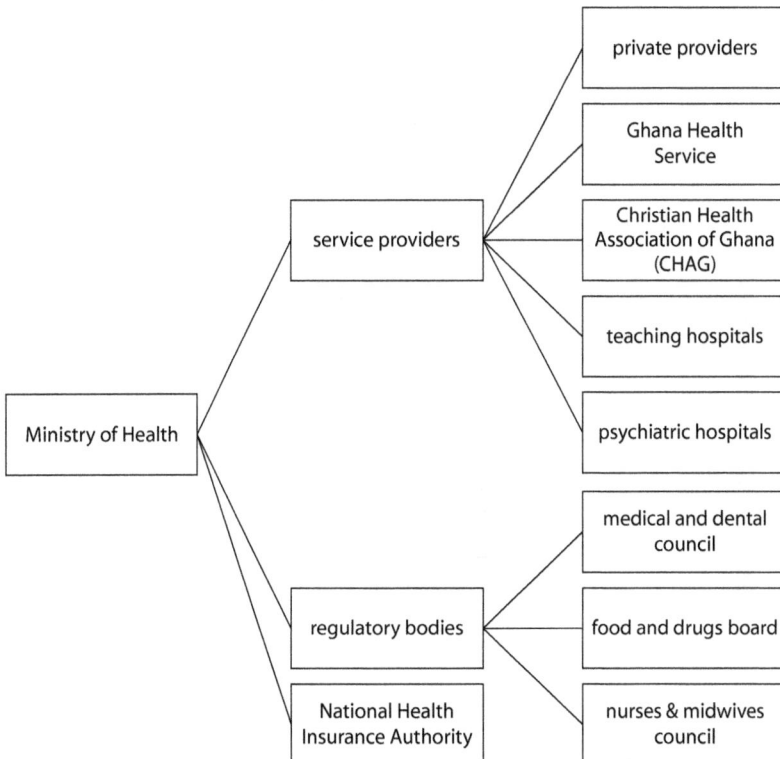

Source: Ministry of Health, modified by World Bank.

Figure 1.4 Ghana's Service Delivery System

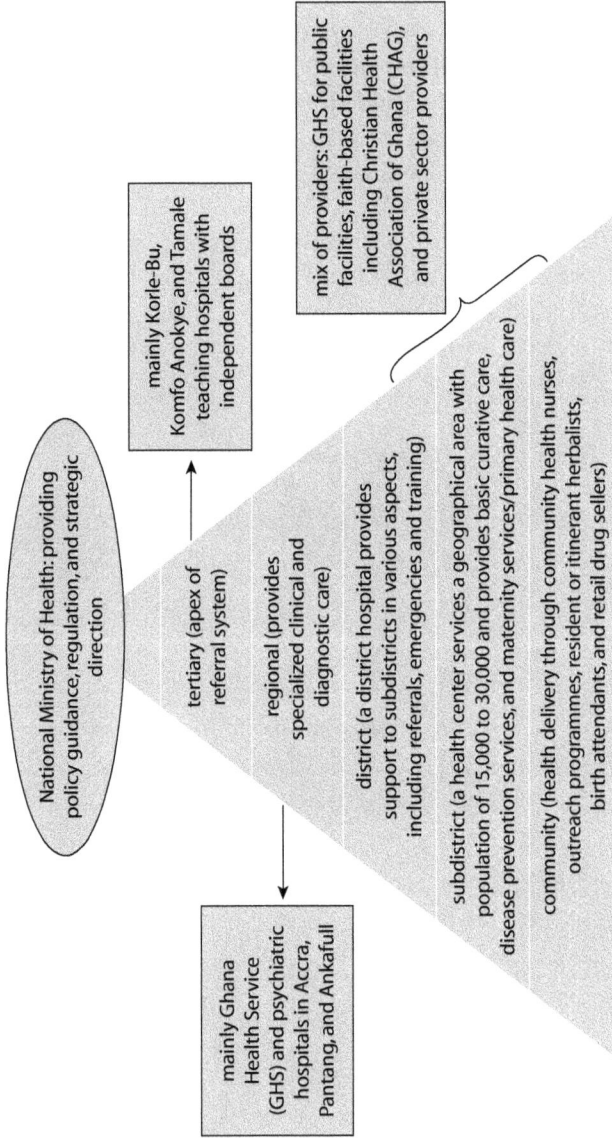

National Ministry of Health: providing policy guidance, regulation, and strategic direction

tertiary (apex of referral system)
- mainly Korle-Bu, Komfo Anokye, and Tamale teaching hospitals with independent boards
- mainly Ghana Health Service (GHS) and psychiatric hospitals in Accra, Pantang, and Ankafull

regional (provides specialized clinical and diagnostic care)

district (a district hospital provides support to subdistricts in various aspects, including referrals, emergencies and training)

subdistrict (a health center services a geographical area with population of 15,000 to 30,000 and provides basic curative care, disease prevention services, and maternity services/primary health care)

community (health delivery through community health nurses, outreach programmes, resident or itinerant herbalists, birth attendants, and retail drug sellers)

mix of providers: GHS for public facilities, faith-based facilities including Christian Health Association of Ghana (CHAG), and private sector providers

Source: Seddoh, Adjei, and Nazzar 2011.

of hospital care in several districts, largely in urban areas. The private sector produces more than half of all services used in virtually every category of the health sector (Sealy, Makinen, and Bitran 2010).

The system also faces many challenges:

- Management, organizational, and distributional problems are serious (Ghana Health Service 2009).
- Increases in critical health sector inputs have not kept pace with population growth or growth in neighboring countries.
- The volume of inputs is lower than in countries with similar levels of income and health spending, and inputs are often used suboptimally, as evidenced by the 60 percent hospital occupancy rate.
- Decentralization has confused roles and responsibilities.

The Manpower, Private Sector, and Infrastructure background papers for the Country Status Report (Saleh forthcoming [2012]) provide in-depth assessments of these service delivery system issues, as does the report by Seddoh, Adjei, and Nazzar (2011) (see also Herbst 2010; Sealy, Makinen, and Bitran 2010; Dubbledam and others 2011; and Saleh forthcoming [2012]). Chapter 3 analyzes these issues.

Functions and Goals of Ghana's Health System and Health Financing

According to the World Health Organization (WHO), the health financing system is one of the six basic building blocks of a health system (the others are service delivery; the health care work force; information; medical products, vaccines, and technologies; and leadership/governance) (figure 1.5). Financing interacts with all of these elements. It has a profound effect on improving health outcomes, ensuring financial protection, and responding to consumers in an equitable, efficient, and sustainable manner.

The three basic health financing functions are raising revenue, pooling risk, and purchasing services (WHO 2000) (figure 1.6). The three critical elements of universal coverage are breadth, scope, and depth (Kutzin, Jakab, and Cashin 2010; WHO 2010).

Countries need to focus on effectively implementing the three health financing functions in order to achieve the basic objectives of improving health outcomes, ensuring financial protection, and responding to consumers in an equitable, efficient, sustainability and sustainable manner.

Figure 1.5   Components and Objectives of a Health System

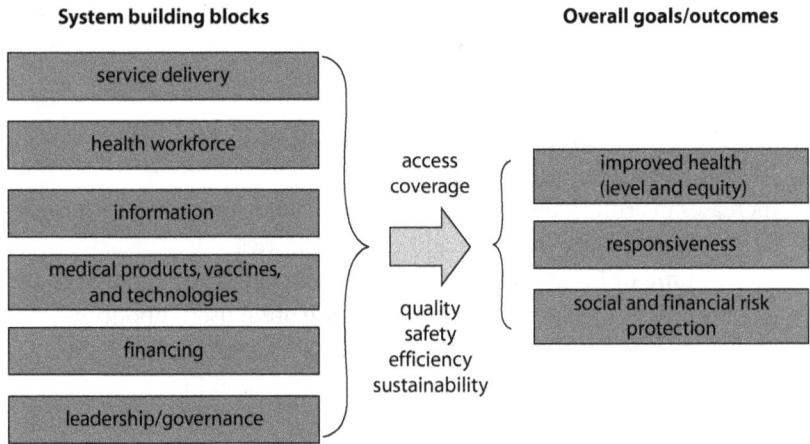

System building blocks   Overall goals/outcomes

service delivery

health workforce   access   improved health
                                          coverage   (level and equity)
information

medical products, vaccines,   responsiveness
and technologies
                                          quality   social and financial risk
financing   safety   protection
                                          efficiency
                                          sustainability
leadership/governance

Source: Adapted from Gottret and Schieber 2006 and WHO 2007.

Figure 1.6   Functions and Goals of Health Financing

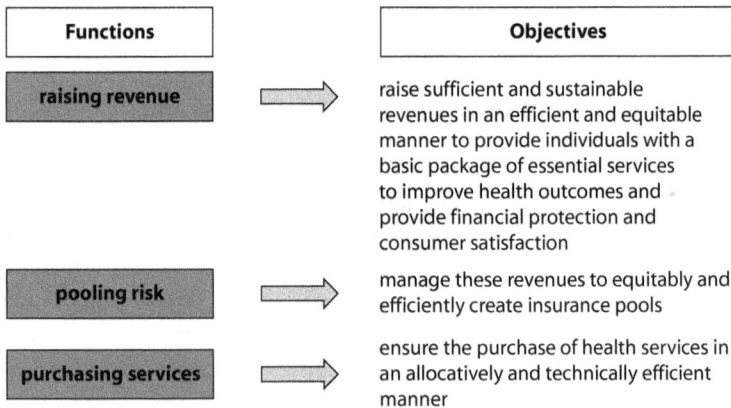

Functions		Objectives
raising revenue	⟹	raise sufficient and sustainable revenues in an efficient and equitable manner to provide individuals with a basic package of essential services to improve health outcomes and provide financial protection and consumer satisfaction
pooling risk	⟹	manage these revenues to equitably and efficiently create insurance pools
purchasing services	⟹	ensure the purchase of health services in an allocatively and technically efficient manner

Source: Gottret and Schieber 2006.

These aspects—equity, efficiency, and sustainability—are sometimes referred to as subgoals of the three basic goals. Neither debates about financing models (such as whether social health insurance or a national health service is a better model) nor ideology-driven "one size fits all" solutions are useful. Instead, policy makers need to focus on the objectives they want to achieve in the context of their underlying demographic, epidemiological, political, geographic, institutional, and economic contexts and design their financing policies to achieve those objectives (see Gottret and Schieber 2006). Doing so will depend on the institutional arrangements and economic incentives embodied in the health financing arrangements and more broadly on the overall health system.

Figure 1.7 provides information about Ghana's transition to universal coverage. According to the NHIS, in 2010, 34 percent of Ghana's population was covered.[2] The scope of the basic benefits package is broad, covering some 95 percent of the burden of disease. The NHIS accounts for only 16 percent of total health expenditures and 30 percent of public health expenditures, however.[3] Out-of-pocket spending accounts for about 37 percent of total health spending, well in excess of the 15–20 percent threshold for adequate financial protection suggested by the WHO. In proposing reforms of Ghana's health financing system, policy makers need to assess the scope, breadth, and depth of coverage. Reform policies must be developed, actuarially estimated, and reconciled with the available fiscal space.

Figure 1.7   Ghana's Transition to Universal Coverage

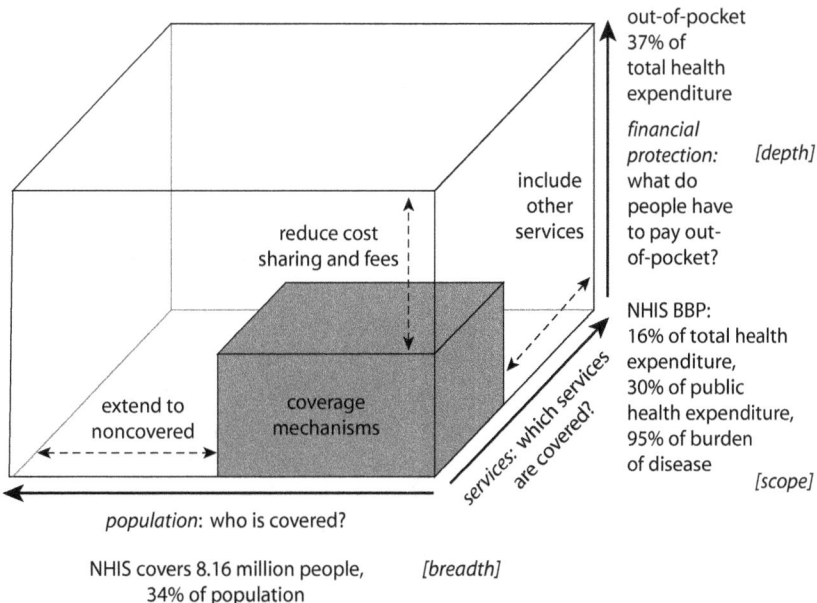

out-of-pocket
37% of
total health
expenditure

*financial
protection:*   *[depth]*
what do
people have
to pay out-
of-pocket?

include
other
services

reduce cost
sharing and fees

NHIS BBP:
16% of total health
expenditure,
30% of public
health expenditure,
95% of burden
of disease
            [scope]

extend to
noncovered

coverage
mechanisms

*services: which services
are covered?*

population: who is covered?

NHIS covers 8.16 million people,   *[breadth]*
34% of population

Source: WHO 2010.

Lack of essential underlying information is a critical problem in Ghana. The last comprehensive National Health Accounts date from 2002; the weights across sources, uses, and service categories used to estimate the latest 2009 National Health Accounts are from this 2002 study, predating the NHIS. Moreover, as Apoya and Marriott (2011) note, no consistently reliable information on NHIS coverage is available.

Ghana's Health Financing System

There is an abundant literature on Ghana's health financing system and the NHIS. The evolution of the system from a classic general revenue–funded national health system (in which free care was provided by the Ministry of Health) to a "cash and carry" system relying on substantial patient payments to a national mandatory health insurance scheme has been well documented (see, for example, NDPC 2009; Durairaj, D'Almeida, and Kirigia 2010; Hendriks 2010; Mensah and others 2010; Nyonator 2010a, 2010b, 2010c; Apoya and Marriott 2011). When it did so, in 2003, Ghana was one of only a handful of low-income countries to enact legislation and earmark significant amounts of funding to establish universal health insurance coverage, provide an extensive basic benefits package with no cost sharing, and begin the transition by covering the poor and other vulnerable populations. Universal coverage in many countries in the Organisation for Economic Co-operation and Development (OECD) grew out of community-based schemes. But these evolutions took place over decades. In contrast, Ghana transitioned its existing community-based health insurance plans to district mutual health insurance schemes, standardized the basic benefits package and administrative procedures, and has basically transitioned these schemes into local branches of the NHIS within just five years, albeit not without problems.

Table 1.1 lays out the governance, administration, membership, provision, and financing arrangements of the NHIS. Seddoh, Adjei, and Nazzar (2011) analyze these features—particularly the administrative, institutional, and operational aspects—in detail. The focus here is on the broader financing, eligibility, benefit, and provider payment issues.

Ghana's achievements have been impressive. But as a country that has just risen from low-income to lower-middle-income status with limited experience in administering health insurance, a complex decentralized administrative structure, an economy open to external shocks, and rapid expansions of enrollment over five years to more than one-third of the

Table 1.1   Features of Ghana's National Health Insurance Scheme

Feature	Description
Legislative instruments	Act 650 (2003) and LI 1809 (2004) are the main legal frameworks guiding the implementation of health insurance in Ghana.
Governance	A 15-member National Health Insurance Council (NHIC) was established to manage the National Health Insurance Fund, provide subsidies to district-wide mutual health insurance schemes, regulate the insurance market, and license and monitor service providers under the scheme.
Administration	A national Health Insurance Secretariat provides administrative support to the NHIC in implementation of the scheme.
	District mutual health insurance schemes (DMHIS), established by sponsors identified by the district assemblies or by the NHIC as corporate bodies, implement the scheme at the district level. Private sector schemes may be established but do not receive government subsidies. They operate as insurance schemes based on a premium, contract, and policy.
	A Health Complaints Committee was established in every district office of the NHIC.
Membership	Enrollment and membership in a DMHIS is mandatory for all residents of Ghana except people in the Ghana Armed Forces or the Ghana Police Service or people who have proof of holding a health insurance policy. People eligible for membership are expected to pay a contribution of GHC 7.20 a year (equivalent to US$7.74 when the act was passed). A period of six months may lapse between payment of membership and issuance of membership cards, which provide access to service. Exemptions from payment are provided to the following groups: • Contributors to the national Social Security and National Insurance Trust (SSNIT) or people drawing pension benefits from the SSNIT. • People under the age of 18 with at least one parent paying membership fees or covered by the exemption clause. • People above the age of 70. • People classified as indigent according to the criteria set by Act 650 and LI 1809.
Service provision	The legislative instrument defines a benefit and an exclusion package for which a member of the scheme may have access.
	Service providers wishing to provide services to members of the scheme have to apply to the NHIC for accreditation and licensing to provide a specified set of services from the benefit package according to their assessed competency.
Financing	Five main sources of funds accrue to a National Health Insurance Fund (NHIF) used primarily to finance services provided and cover administrative costs of the NHIC:

(continued next page)

Table 1.1   *(continued)*

Feature	Description
	• appropriation of 2.5% of all funds mobilized from workers' pension contributions to the SSNIT
	• an ad valorem tax of 2.5% levied specifically for health insurance on all goods and services purchased or provided on which value added tax is charged
	• government annual budgetary allocations proposed and approved by parliament to the NHIF
	• accruals from investments of surplus funds held in the NHIF by the NHIC
	• gifts and donations made by individuals or organizations to the NHIF

Source: Authors, based on Act 650 (2003) and LI 1809 (2004).
Note: Contributions paid for membership do not accrue to the NHIF for reallocation in support of service provision. They are held at the district level for administrative support at that level.

population (according to the NHIS estimate), the NHIS has encountered serious growing pains and now finds itself at an important crossroad. The diversified funding sources for the NHIS are proving to be relatively stable and, as shown in chapter 4, are likely to be a viable financing base for the scheme over the next three to five years. However, revenue will not be sufficient to sustain the NHIS under its current expenditure patterns and expansion plans. Unless the structural inefficiencies in the NHIS and in the health service delivery system are addressed, the NHIS is projected to become insolvent by as early as 2013. It is difficult to argue for bringing additional resources into such a highly inefficient system. The NHIS needs to undertake major structural reforms to fundamentally alter its expenditure patterns in order to ensure its financial sustainability, effectively serve the Ghanaian people, and become a successful African and international model of good practice.

Analysis of these issues requires an understanding of the flows of funds in Ghana's health system (figure 1.8). Revenues for the system come from nontax revenues, taxes, donor contributions, and out-of-pocket payments by individuals. Funds are earmarked for the NHIS from the budget, but the budget also supports the Ministry of Health, and some of the earmarked funding to NHIS is passed through to the Ministry of Health. Donor funds provide direct support to the government, the NHIS, and the Ministry of Health.

A background note prepared for this report shows that financial resources and expenditures for health for both the Ministry of Health and

Figure 1.8   Flows of Funds in Ghana's Health System

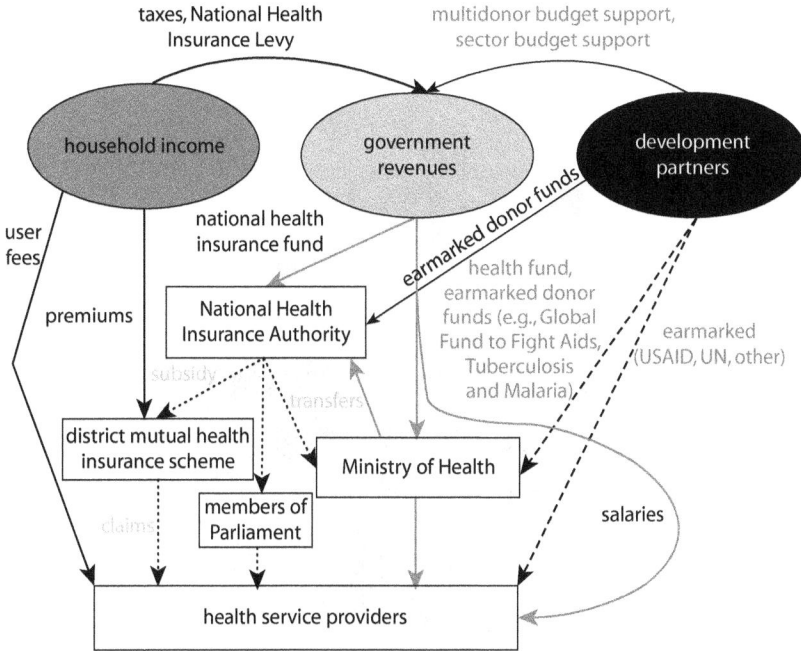

Source: Adapted from Appiah-Denkyira, Nartey, and Enemark 2005.

the NHIS increased substantially between 2005 and 2009 (El Idrissi 2011). In nominal terms, according to Ministry of Health financial statements, ministry expenditures increased from $349 million in 2005 to $786 million in 2009, and the expenditures of the NHIS (excluding transfers to Ministry of Health and payments to Ministry of Health facilities in order to avoid double-counting) increased from $13 million to $181 million.[4]

Figures 1.9 and 1.10 from this background note display the Ministry of Health's sources of revenues. They reveal the increasing importance of NHIS transfers and the decreasing importance of direct government appropriations. In addition to the direct NHIS transfers to the Ministry of Health, ministry facilities themselves are becoming increasingly dependent on internally generated funds, which consist of out-of-pocket payments and direct NHIS insurance payments (figure 1.11). In 2009, internally generated funds accounted for about one-quarter of public provider revenue. These direct transfers to the Ministry of Health and the increasing dependence of public health care providers on NHIS revenues

Figure 1.9   Sources of Ministry of Health Revenues, 2005–09

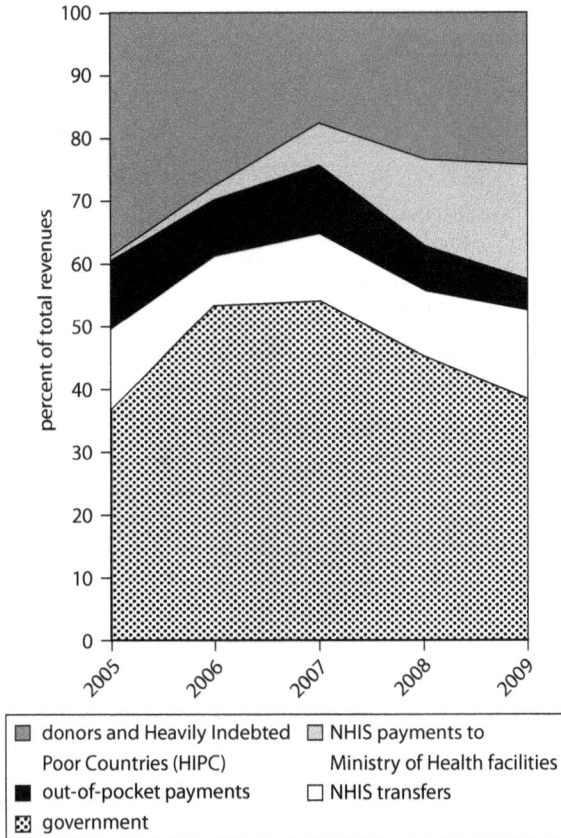

Source: Ministry of Health 2011.

raise important questions about whether NHIS is purely an insurance/
purchasing entity or whether it is increasingly being required to take on
the roles of the Ministry of Health/Ghana Health System and the private
sector in developing the capacity of the health system. The increasing size
of these transfers has major implications for the sustainability of the
NHIS, as discussed below. The impact of the NHIS as the single national
insurer and purchaser is very large and continues to grow.

The strategic purchasing function of the NHIS is maturing. Although
it has not yet exploited its purchasing power as the single unified
national health insurance entity, the NHIS has the potential to be a force

Figure 1.10   Sources of Ministry of Health Revenues, 2009

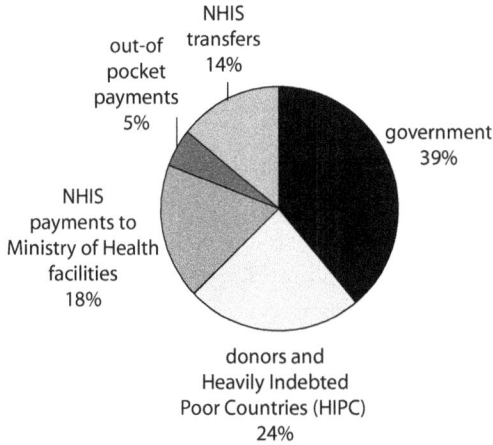

NHIS
transfers
14%

out-of
pocket
payments
5%

government
39%

NHIS
payments to
Ministry of Health
facilities
18%

donors and
Heavily Indebted
Poor Countries (HIPC)
24%

Source: Ministry of Health 2011.

Figure 1.11   Funds Generated Internally by Ministry of Health Facilities, 2005–09

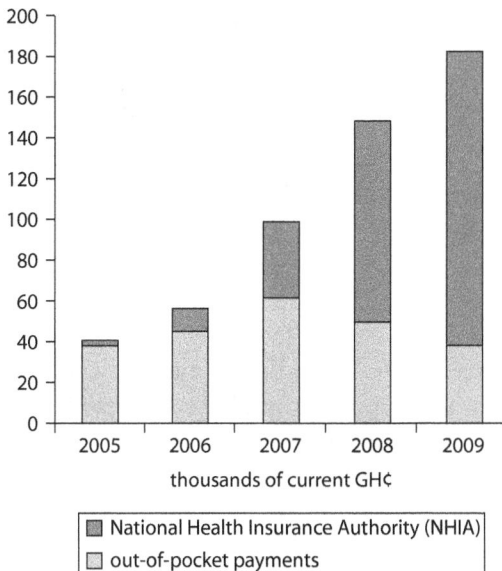

thousands of current GH¢

■ National Health Insurance Authority (NHIA)
□ out-of-pocket payments

Source: Ministry of Health 2011.

for change and modernization in service delivery. In particular, it has made an ongoing effort to modernize its provider payment systems and use this purchasing tool more effectively to achieve broader objectives for the system.

Regulation 37(2) L.I. 1809 of the health insurance legislative framework requires the NHIA to develop uniform provider payment mechanisms to reimburse accredited providers for services rendered to NHIS subscribers. The provider payment mechanisms suggested in the law include capitation, fee-for-service, and other mechanisms, as determined by the NHIA. Initially, the NHIA adopted an itemized fee-for-service payment system, paying providers for each service rendered. In addition to the natural incentive of fee-for-service payment to increase utilization with no lever to contain costs, the tariffs used by different schemes were not uniform. Inequities emerged as different facilities were reimbursed at different rates for treating the same condition.

In response to the challenges of the itemized fee-for-service system, the NHIA implemented Ghana Diagnosis Related Groups (G-DRGs) in 2008. DRGs are standard groupings of diseases that are clinically similar, require comparable treatments or operations, and use similar health care resources. Under the G-DRG payment system, providers are reimbursed the same fixed tariff for cases that fall into the same diagnostic category. There are about 550 G-DRGs, including bundled payment for outpatient services.

The G-DRG system has been fully implemented. Although challenges remain, the payment system is functioning well, understood, and generally accepted by providers. The payment system has not, however, succeeded in containing costs or driving efficiencies in service delivery, particularly for outpatient services, which accounted for 70 percent of NHIS claims and 30 percent of total costs in 2009. Between 2007 and 2009, the value of the average outpatient claim increased by nearly 50 percent, from $6.93 to $10.11.

By 2010, the NHIA was faced with concerns about unchecked cost escalation, apparent supplier-induced demand, and little evidence of improved quality or effectiveness of services. After careful consideration of the challenges, it decided to pilot a capitation payment system for primary care services in the Ashanti region in 2011. The Ashanti region has a population of more than 3.8 million people and accounts for nearly 25 percent of total NHIS claims. It is hoped that the pilot will help orient the NHIS toward making more effective use of provider payment mechanisms and begin to address more fundamental problems in the service

Figure 1.12   Projected Revenues and Expenditures of Ghana's National Health Insurance Scheme, 2008–18

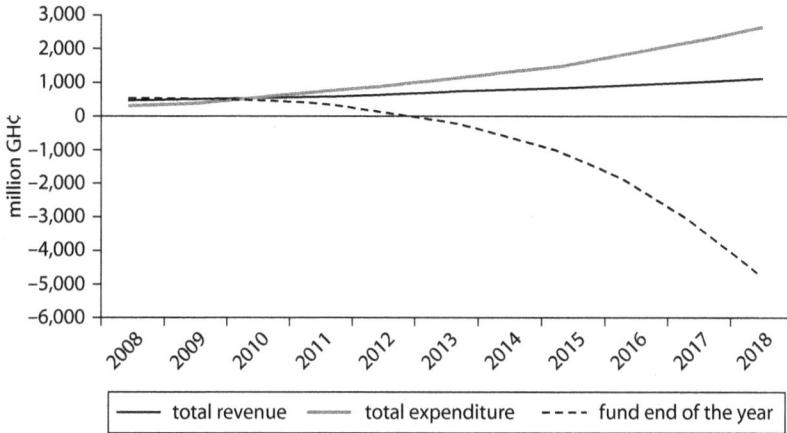

Sources: NHIA 2009; World Bank 2011.

delivery system, such as the lack of focus on prevention, poorly coordinated care, and inadequate management of chronic diseases.

Figure 1.12 displays the income and expenditure cash flows of the NHIS. In 2009, 61 percent of NHIS income was derived from the National Health Insurance Levy (NHIL), the 2.5 percentage point value added tax earmark; another 15.5 percent came from the 2.5 percentage points of the 18.5 percent Social Security National Insurance Trust (SSNIT) contributions levied on formal sector workers and their employers.[5] Premium income accounted for less than 4 percent of income (this figure is likely to be an underestimate, as premiums are paid directly to the district schemes and often do not show up in NHIS records).

As the NHIS accounts for some 30–40 percent of all public spending on health in Ghana—and its share is increasing rapidly—ensuring its efficiency and sustainability is a major national priority. However, money alone does not tell the story: it is value for money in terms of health outcomes, financial protection, and consumer responsiveness that matters. Chapter 2 assesses the performance of Ghana's health system.

Notes

1. The NHIS is the term used to describe the health insurance system as a whole. The National Health Insurance Authority (NHIA) is the managing

body for the NHIS. The National Health Insurance Fund (NHIF) is the statutory fund in which resources to fund the NHIS accumulate.

2. Apoya and Marriott (2011) claim that Ghana's NHIS covered only 18 percent of the population in 2009; the NHIS claimed that more than 60 percent of the population was covered. In response to these large disparities, the NHIS revised its methodology for estimating coverage. According to its 2010 annual report, the number of "active" members was 8.16 million in 2010, or 34 percent of the population (NHIS 2011).

3. If one uses 2009 expenditure data from the 2010 NHIS annual report on contributions from social insurance organizations instead of National Health Accounting data from the WHO and applies this figure to the WHO 2009 estimate of total and government health expenditures for Ghana, NHIS accounts for 24 percent of total health spending and 45 percent of all government spending. The large disparity in these figures underscores the critical need for better information. The WHO uses data from Ghana's last comprehensive National Health Accounting (2002) to estimate sources and uses of funds in its national health account estimates. It is critical that Ghana conduct a new comprehensive National Health Accounting and that the NHIS continue refining its methodology and data for deriving its coverage figures.

4. There are serious data inconsistencies between the National Health Accounts estimate by the WHO and expenditure information obtained from administrative records. Ghana has not conducted a full-blown National Health Accounting since 2002. Administrative records are also problematic given the poor, albeit improving, state of Ghana's public sector management and Health Management Information System (see El-Idrissi 2011 and chapter 3 of this report).

5. The 2009 NHIA data were used here rather than the recently released 2010 data because the performance assessments in chapter 2 are based on 2009 information (the latest currently available) and the detailed 2009 information on sources of funding and expenditures was available in Hendriks' (2010) actuarial report but not in the 2010 NHIA report.

References

Apoya, P., and A. Marriott. 2011. *Achieving a Shared Goal: Free Universal Health Care in Ghana*. Alliance for Reproductive Health Rights, Essential Services Platform of Ghana, Integrated Social Development Centre and Oxfam International, United Kingdom.

Appiah, E., C. Herbst, A. Soucat, and K. Saleh, eds. Forthcoming. *Towards Interventions on Human Resources for Health in Ghana: Evidence for Health Workforce Planning and Results*. Washington, DC: World Bank.

Appiah-Denkyira, E., A. Nartey, and U. Enemark. 2005. *Review of Financing Strategy and Resource Allocation Criteria*. Ministry of Health, Accra.

Benzing, C., and C. Hung. 2009. "A Comparison of the Motivations of Small Business Owners in Africa." *Journal of Small Business and Enterprise Development* 16 (1): 60–77.

Dubbeldam, R., P. Asman, C. Cuninghame, R. McGreghor, and P. K. Mensah. 2011. *Country Status Report: Health Infrastructure Management Draft*. World Bank, Washington, DC.

Durairaj, V., S. D'Almeida, and J. Kirigia. 2010. *Ghana's Approach to Social Health Protection*. Background paper for the 2010 World Health Report, World Health Organization, Geneva.

El Idrissi, M. 2011. "Background Note on Health Expenditures in Ghana." World Bank, Dakar, Senegal.

Ghana Health Service. 2009. *The Health Sector in Ghana Facts and Figures 2009*. Accra.

Ghana Statistical Service and WIEGO (Woman in Informal Employment: Globalizing and Organizing). 2005. "The Informal Economy in Ghana: A Comparative Perspective." Paper presented at the conference cohosted by the Ghana Statistical Service and WIEGO, Accra, October 24.

Gottret, P., and G. Schieber. 2006. *Health Financing Revisited*. World Bank, Washington, DC.

Hendriks, R. 2010. "National Health Insurance Ghana". World Bank, Washington, DC, and Ghana Ministry of Health, Accra.

Herbst, C. 2010. *Country Status Report: Human Resources for Health in Ghana*. Ghana Ministry of Health, Accra, and World Bank, Washington, DC.

Kutzin, J., M. Jakab, and C. Cashin. 2010. "Lessons from Health Financing Reform in Eastern Europe and the Former Soviet Union." *Health Economics, Policy and Law* 5 (2): 135–47.

Mensah, J., J. Oppong, K. Bobi-Barimah, G. Frempong, and W. Sabi. 2010. *An Evaluation of the Ghana National Health Insurance Scheme in the Context of the Health MDGs*. Global Development Network.

Ministry of Health. 2011. *Health Sector Medium Term Development Plan 2010–2013*. Accra.

NDPC (National Development Planning Commission). 2009. *2008 Citizens' Assessment of the National Health Insurance Scheme*. Accra.

NHIA (National Health Insurance Authority). 2009. *Annual Report 2009*. Accra.

NHIS (National Health Insurance Scheme). 2011. *2010 Annual Report*. Accra.

Nyonator, F. 2010a. "District Mutual Health Insurance Scheme Operations in Ghana: Key Operational Components, Quality Assurance and Challenges." PowerPoint presentation, World Bank Institute, Washington, DC.

————. 2010b. "Establishment and Governance of the National Health Insurance Scheme (NHIS) Based on District Mutual Health Insurance Schemes." PowerPoint presentation, World Bank Institute, Washington, DC.

————. 2010c. *Ghana Case Study*. World Bank Institute Health Reform Flagship Course, Washington, DC.

Saleh, Karima. Forthcoming (2012). *The Health Sector in Ghana: A Comprehensive Assessment*. Washington, DC: World Bank.

Sealy, S., M. Makinen, and R. Bitran. 2010. *Country Assessment of the Private Health Sector in Ghana*. Washington, DC: Results for Development.

Seddoh, A., S. Adjei, and A. Nazzar. 2011. *Ghana's National Health Insurance Scheme*. Rockefeller Foundation, New York.

World Bank. 2011. *Republic of Ghana: Joint Review of Public Expenditure and Financial Management*. Africa Region, Washington, DC.

WHO (World Health Organization). 2000. *Health Systems: Improving Performance*. Geneva: World Health Organization.

————. 2007. *Strengthening Health Systems to Improve Health Outcomes*. Geneva: World Health Organization.

————. 2008. *The Global Burden of Disease 2004 Update*. Geneva: World Health Organization.

————. 2010. *Health Systems Financing: The Path to Universal Coverage*. Geneva: World Health Organization.

CHAPTER 2

Ghana's Health Financing: A Performance Assessment

Among the small number of low- and middle-income countries that have enacted legislation and begun the transition to universal health insurance coverage, Ghana is one of the few countries in Africa to begin by publically financing care to the poor and other vulnerable groups. It has done so by imposing a payroll tax on public and private formal sector employees, obtaining subsidized premiums from informal sector workers, and earmarking 2.5 percentage points of the country's value added tax (VAT) to help support the system. The purpose of the universal health insurance reform is to improve health outcomes, provide financial protection, ensure equity, and be responsive to consumers while achieving long-run financial sustainability.

Legislation authorizing Ghana's national health financing reform was passed in 2003 and 2004, and implementation started in 2005. Since then it has been evolving from community-based health insurance plans (mutuals and for-profit) to a system of district mutual health insurance schemes (DMHISs) subject to a standard set of rules under a National Health Insurance Administration (NHIA) to a national system in which the local DMHISs are in the process of becoming branches of the NHIA. The system has made progress in increasing coverage, standardizing administration, and developing and beginning implementation of a modern Health Management Information System (HMIS) and provider payment mechanism.

This chapter assesses the performance of Ghana's health system in terms of three measures:

- changes over time in Ghana and relative to relevant African comparators in health outcomes (under-five mortality, maternal mortality, and life expectancy); delivery system capacity (number of beds, physicians, total health workers); total, public, and private health spending; and for the latest available year (generally 2009), benchmarking Ghana's performance relative to similar income and health spending global comparator countries
- financial protection, equity, and benefit incidence by income class
- consumer satisfaction and responsiveness

The analysis builds on studies of health spending, inputs, outcomes, and household spending, (NDPC 2009; WHO 2011; IMF 2011a, IMF 2011b; World Bank 2011a, 2011b, 2012). It undertakes for the first time an extensive international benchmarking analysis; assesses changes over time in the financial protection/equity of the system at both the macro and micro levels; and analyzes the consumer responsiveness of the system.

There is no simple metric for analyzing the performance of a health system—and even if such a metric existed, reliable aggregate indexes (of health outcomes, financial protection, consumer responsiveness, equity, efficiency, and sustainability) are not widely available. Moreover, it is extremely difficult to assess the complex interactions among all relevant performance determinants of health systems and other relevant systems (such as education and sanitation), including demand-side factors (see OECD 2010; WHO 2010).

Assessing changes over time in health sector outcomes, inputs, and spending and comparing these components across countries with similar income and health spending provides some crude measures for assessing relative performance. Countries that have better health and financial protection outcomes, report higher levels of consumer responsiveness, use fewer inputs, and achieve outcomes at lower spending levels are worthy of in-depth analysis as "good practice" cases (see Gottret, Schieber, and Waters 2008).

This chapter is organized as follows. The first section summarizes trends in outcomes, inputs, and spending over time. The second section uses household-level information to analyze equity in terms of utilization, insurance coverage, and financial protection against impoverishment. The last section examines consumer responsiveness. The annex provides a time series analysis of trends in outcomes, inputs, and spending as well as comparisons for 2009 of Ghana against other countries with similar levels of income.

Health Outcomes, Inputs, and Health Spending

Trends in health outcomes and inputs are analyzed for 1960–2009; health spending is analyzed for 1995–2009. Ghana's performance is then compared with that of other countries for each measure based on the latest year of data available (generally 2009).

Health Outcomes

Ghana achieved some impressive improvements in health outcomes between 1960 and 2009, but challenges remain:

- Under-five mortality decreased from 218 in 1960 to 77 per 1,000 live births in 2009. But relative to other countries with comparable income and health spending globally, Ghana has high under-five mortality. Achieving the Millennium Development Goal (MDG) target of reducing under-five mortality by two-thirds between 1990 and 2015 will be difficult.
- Maternal mortality decreased from 630 in 1990 to 350 per 100,000 live births in 2008. But relative to other countries with comparable income and health spending, Ghana's maternal mortality ratio is high. Like many Sub-Saharan African countries, Ghana is unlikely to achieve the MDG target of reducing maternal mortality by three-quarters between 1990 and 2015.
- Life expectancy increased from 46.0 years in 1960 to 63.4 years in 2009. In 2009, Ghana had higher life expectancy than other countries with comparable income and health spending.

Health Inputs

The number of hospital beds and health sector personnel in Ghana have been increasing since 1960, although trends in the past 20 years have been somewhat more erratic:

- Ghana's physician to population ratio increased from 0.05 per 1,000 in 1960 to 0.09 in 2009. Although Ghana was in the mid-range among comparator countries in 1960 and its ratio increased significantly over this period, in 2009 it still had fewer physicians per capita than countries with comparable income and health spending.

- Relative to comparators, Ghana had fewer skilled birth attendants and fewer total health workers per capita.
- The number of hospital beds increased from 0.78 in 1960 to 0.93 per 1,000 people in 2009. The ratio has been declining since 1985, however, a trend also seen in some African comparator countries. In 2009, Ghana had fewer beds per capita than countries with comparable income and health spending.

Ghana appears to have less hospital infrastructure and manpower than other comparable income and health spending countries. If inputs were being used efficiently, lower levels of inputs could be viewed as positive. However, given Ghana's relatively poor health outcomes and near average spending levels (assessed below), an in-depth assessment of the health system's infrastructure, including its distribution, utilization levels, governance, and quality, is needed to better understand its performance. Micro studies of technical efficiency are also needed. Such an assessment is undertaken in the Ghana Country Status Report (Saleh forthcoming [2012]) and in chapter 3 of this report.

Health Spending

Health spending can be measured in various ways, each of which provides complementary information about performance. One can analyze spending in terms of total, public, private, or out-of-pocket spending; in local currency units or some numeraire currency, such as U.S. dollars (based on exchange rates) or international dollars (based on purchasing power parity); in nominal or real terms; in terms of total or per capita spending; and relative to overall gross domestic product (GDP) and total government spending.

Annex 2A presents an extensive analysis of all of these measures. It presents time series data on selected African comparators for 1995–2009 as well as comparisons of Ghana with global comparators (countries with similar levels of income and health spending) for 2009. Key findings include the following:

- Both total and per capita health spending increased significantly in Ghana between 1995 and 2009. In dollar terms, per capita health spending doubled, from $27 to $54. In terms of purchasing power parity, per capita spending rose from $63 to $125.
- The composition of health spending changed. As a share of total health expenditure, public spending in Ghana increased from 44 percent to

53 percent, private spending decreased from 56 percent to 47 percent, and out-of-pocket spending decreased from 44 percent to 37 percent.

- The share of GDP Ghana devoted to health dropped from 5.3 percent in 1995 to 4.9 percent in 2009. Total health spending increased 3 percent more rapidly than GDP (nominal elasticity of 1.03), public spending increased 13 percent more rapidly (nominal elasticity of 1.13), and private spending increased 7 percent less rapidly (nominal elasticity of 0.93). These increases were smaller than the averages for Sub-Saharan Africa (nominal elasticities of 1.09 for total health spending, 1.17 of public spending, and 1.02 for private spending). After implementation of the National Health Insurance Scheme (NHIS) in 2005, total health spending increased at the same rate as GDP (nominal elasticity of 1.00), public spending continued to increase significantly more rapidly than GDP (nominal elasticity of 1.11), and private spending grew less rapidly than GDP (nominal elasticity of 0.87).

- Relative to total government spending, government spending on health increased 12 percent a year faster than overall government spending over 1995–2009 (nominal elasticity of 1.12), but only 2.1 percent faster over 2004–09 (nominal elasticity of 1.02). Relative to total government revenues, government health spending increased 1 percent a year faster over 1995–2009 (nominal elasticity of 1.01) and 15 percent a year faster over 2004–09 (nominal elasticity of 1.15). These figures reflect the fluctuations in public spending, revenues, and GDP as a result of both exogenous global factors, such as the global financial crisis and aid flows, and the government's decision to implement the NHIS and grant large salary increases to doctors.

As a result of revisions to its GDP in 2010, Ghana was elevated to the ranks of lower-middle-income countries. Its position in 2009 with respect to other lower-middle-income countries can be summarized as follows:

- Total health spending as a share of GDP (4.9 percent) was slightly below the global average for countries at this level of income. Per capita spending (of $54 based in U.S. dollars and $125 in international dollars) was about average.
- Measured as shares of total health spending (53 percent) and total government spending (12.6 percent), public spending on health in

Ghana was well above the global average for countries with comparable levels of income. As a share of GDP (2.6 percent), public spending on health was about average, as were public spending on health per capita levels ($29 in U.S. dollars, $66 in international dollars). Before the 2010 GDP revision, Ghana's public spending on health was above the average of its global comparators on most of these measures. Like many other African comparators, however, Ghana did not reach the Abuja target of dedicating 15 percent of the government budget to health.

• Private spending as a share of total health spending (47 percent) and GDP (2.3 percent), as well as in per capita spending ($25 in U.S. dollars, $59 in international dollars) were close to the global averages for countries with comparable levels of income.

• Annual out-of-pocket spending ($20 in U.S. dollars, $46 in international dollars) accounted for 79 percent of all private and 37 percent of total health spending in Ghana—far higher than the 15–20 percent out-of-pocket criterion of the World Health Organization (WHO). It was at or slightly above the average for countries with comparable levels of income, indicating that financial protection is about average or slightly worse.

• Ghana's revenue to GDP ratio (13.5 percent) was well below the levels in other countries with comparable levels of income. External aid as a share of total health spending (14.0 percent) was average. There is concern, however, that donors may reduce their very significant levels of assistance to Ghana in response to the increased revenue from new oil production, the global financial crisis, and Ghana's newfound lower-middle-income country status.

Global comparisons of health spending using the revised GDP figures and the latest National Health Accounting data suggest that Ghana's overall level of health spending relative to GDP was slightly below the average for countries with comparable levels of income. Its public share was above average, and its out-of-pocket spending was at or slightly above that of its global comparators.

Continuing to expand coverage may be challenging, given Ghana's low revenue effort. There is also the question of whether Ghana's globally average but still sizable share of external assistance will continue. Ghana's relatively weak outcomes on health and financial protection—two key goals of health systems—and low levels of inputs raise serious questions about allocative and technical efficiency. The next section analyzes household-level information in order to explore financial protection and equity issues and gain a better understanding of the impact of the NHIS on access to essential services and health outcomes.

Equity and Financial Protection

Household-level consumption and expenditure data were available through 2006; household-level wealth data were available only for 2008. It is critical for the government to obtain more recent household consumption and expenditure information so that it can assess the impact of the NHIS on equity and financial protection, both currently and over time.

Equity in accessing NHIS coverage was examined by looking at both registration and cardholder status by wealth quintile. Equity in health care utilization was assessed by analyzing differences in utilization rates across wealth quintiles, before and after introduction of the NHIS. Overall health care utilization as well as utilization of maternity services, a high priority in Ghana, were also studied.

Survey microdata are needed to estimate equity and financial protection indicators. Ghana conducts three major surveys: the Ghana Living Standard Survey (GLSS), conducted in 2005/2006; the Ghana Demographic and Health Survey for 2003 and 2008; and the 2008 Citizens' Assessment Survey of the National Development Planning Commission. Of these surveys, only the GLSS 2005/2006 collected data on household income and expenditure, which are needed to estimate financial protection indicators. Because implementation of the NHIS was just starting in 2005, however, the GLSS was not able to capture differences in patterns of utilization among insured and uninsured. In view of this limitation, this study relied on the other two surveys, which do not include income and expenditure data. The missing data were estimated using a wealth index, based on assets households own. These data were disaggregated by the NHIS status of respondents. The incidence of both benefits and financing of health spending by income quintile was also examined, based on a study by Akazili, Gyapong, and McIntyre (2011) and a World Bank report (World Bank 2012) on health equity and financial protection in Ghana.

Coverage

Table 2.1 shows the percentages of men and women 15–49 years old with NHIS registrations and NHIS cards in the highest and lowest wealth quintiles. (The differences between registration and cardholder status have to do with waiting periods and administrative processing times between registration and card receipt.)

The percentage of men and woman that are registered with the NHIS and hold NHIS cards is larger in the top wealth quintile than in the bottom wealth quintile. The differences are striking: 20 percent of men in the top quintile have NHIS cards, compared with only 10 percent of men in the bottom quintile. Among women, 29 percent in the top quintile and 17 percent in the bottom quintile hold NHIS cards. The registration figures show similar disparities.

This pattern is particularly troublesome given the extensive granting of exemptions from premiums for various groups, including the poor. It would appear that both the definition of indigence and outreach activities to ensure enrollment of the most vulnerable people need to be reassessed.

Health Care Utilization

Health care utilization in Ghana fluctuated over the past 15 years. In the early 1990s, 51 percent of the population reported having forgone care during illness or injury. This figure climbed to 56 percent in 1998 (63 percent among the poor). The decline seems to have abated, as seen in improvements in utilization patterns as of 2005 (table 2.2). Marked improvements in utilization of pharmacists and hospitals were observed among all groups, even the poor.

Table 2.1   Coverage of National Health Insurance Scheme, by Gender and Wealth Quintile, 2008

(percentage of Ghanaians 15–49 years old covered)

Gender/wealth quintile	Registered with the NHIS	Hold NHIS card
Women		
Lowest 20 percent	29	17
Highest 20 percent	47	29
Men		
Lowest 20 percent	17	10
Highest 20 percent	38	20

Source: GSS, GHS, and ICF Macro 2009.

Table 2.2   Facility Consulted in Ghana in Case of Illness or Injury, 1991–2006
(percent of respondents)

Facility	1991/92			1998/99			2005/06		
	Poor	Nonpoor	All	Poor	Nonpoor	All	Poor	Nonpoor	All
Hospital	13.7	22.6	18.6	8.6	18.7	15.0	12.2	21.5	19.5
Pharmacy	1.7	5.0	3.5	1.4	3.9	3.0	22.7	20.3	20.8
Other	26.8	27.3	27.1	26.9	25.2	25.8	19.6	19.6	19.6
Did not consult	57.8	45.1	50.8	63.2	52.2	56.2	45.6	38.6	40.1

Source: World Bank 2011a.

This study used the most recent data, the 2008 Citizens' Assessment Survey from the National Development Planning Commission, to examine utilization patterns of the insured versus the uninsured. Among people who reported getting ill or injured in the four weeks before the survey, people with insurance were more likely to go to a formal health facility (table 2.3). Being insured had the strongest effect on utilization of health facilities for the lowest quintile. The largest difference was in the utilization of government hospitals, which 39 percent of people with insurance and just 12 percent of the uninsured used when ill or injured.

When uninsured individuals become ill or injured, many resort to self-medication: 32.5 percent of the uninsured went directly to a pharmacy (table 2.4). In contrast, only 7.0 percent of the insured self-medicated. The same trend is seen among people who forgo treatment: 9.9 percent of the uninsured did not seek care, compared with 2.6 percent of the insured. The highest utilization rates for going to an herbal healer, self-medicating, and forgoing treatment were among the uninsured in the poorest quintile.

Between 2003 and 2008, more women began to shift toward facility-based deliveries: the share of home deliveries declined from 53 percent in 2003 to 42 percent in 2008 (table 2.5). Even women from the bottom two quintiles started to give birth in health facilities, especially government-owned facilities.

The same trend is observed in delivery assistance, where skilled birth attendance gained ground (table 2.6). The highest rates of increase in utilization were with a medical doctor, particularly for women in the second wealth quintile (among whom utilization rates almost doubled) and women in the third quintile (among whom utilization rates more than tripled). Women in these two quintiles also exhibited a modest increase in assistance by nurses and midwives during delivery. As a result of these increases, utilization of services for traditional birth attendants and relatives decreased for all quintiles except the lowest.

Table 2.3 Percent of Ill/Injured in Ghana Who Sought Care at a Health Facility, by Wealth Quintile and Insurance Status, 2008

Wealth quintile	Government hospital		Government health center		Mission hospital		Private hospital		Private clinic	
	Insured	Uninsured	Insured	Uninsured	Insured	Uninsured	Insured	Uninsured	Insured	Uninsured
Lowest	39.2	11.9	35.3	24.9	7.2	1.4	1.6	1.3	2.2	0
Second	38.8	12.6	28.9	25.6	5.8	0.80	2.2	2.3	5.4	4.9
Middle	33.5	36.5	37.4	15.5	5.8	3.1	2.3	10.0	5.1	6.7
Fourth	39.3	24.9	19.2	10.0	5.7	5.3	3.1	4.5	12.6	6.5
Highest	42.0	31.9	14.2	8.7	6.6	3.2	15.5	12.0	10.3	12.1
Total	38.6	22.0	26.3	17.9	6.2	2.6	5.3	3.8	7.4	5.5

Source: Authors' calculation, based on data from NDPC 2009.

Table 2.4   Percent of Ill/Injured in Ghana Who Self-Treated or Sought Care at a Nonformal Facility, by Wealth Quintile and Insurance Status, 2008

Wealth quintile	Drugstore		Herbal healer		Other facilities		Forgo treatment	
	Insured	Uninsured	Insured	Uninsured	Insured	Uninsured	Insured	Uninsured
Lowest	5.1	30.7	2.7	7.4	0.9	0.0	2.9	20.0
Second	6.3	38.6	1.4	3.0	1.3	0.8	5.0	10.4
Middle	6.8	28.0	0.9	1.1	0.0	0.0	2.4	7.0
Fourth	7.9	40.7	0.0	0.0	0.0	0.0	3.0	3.3
Highest	8.4	21.2	0.7	0.0	0.9	0.0	0.0	5.4
Total	7.0	32.5	1.1	2.7	0.6	0.2	2.6	9.9

Source: Authors' calculation, based on data from NDPC 2009.

Pregnant women from all but the bottom wealth quintile appear to have good access to prenatal and delivery care services, regardless of insurance status. Most pregnant women sought delivery assistance from skilled birth attendants (table 2.7) and delivered in health facilities (table 2.8). The effect of insurance on reducing the probability of delivering at home was greatest for women in the lowest quintiles (more than a 20 percentage point difference for the three lowest quintiles).

Women in the lowest wealth quintile continued to give birth at home without a trained birth attendant, even if they had insurance. Ensuring their access to maternal care services thus appears to require more than just health insurance. There would appear to be some scope to improve the reach of community health workers, introduced by the Ghana Health Service in 2003. Their primary responsibility is to provide services in the community-based health planning and services (CHPS) zones. Their responsibilities should be broadened to ensure that women in the lowest quintile are made aware of the importance of maternal care protocols.

For the top four quintiles, the focus should be on ensuring that pregnant women seek prenatal care during the first trimester of pregnancy, as the WHO recommends. On average, the first prenatal care check-up in Ghana is delayed until early in the second trimester (figure 2.1).

Out-of-Pocket Payments and Financial Protection

The most recent data on out-of-pocket payments and poverty come from the 2005/2006 Ghana Living Standards Survey. These data suggest that the burden of health payments appears to be relatively low in Ghana, although households in the poorest consumption quintile allocate a larger share of expenditures to health care than do wealthier households. Households in the lowest consumption quintile spent about 3.2 percent

Table 2.5 Percent of Pregnant Women in Ghana Who Delivered in a Health Facility, 2003 and 2008

Wealth quintile	Public sector facility		Private sector facility		Home		Other		Missing data		Number of births	
	2003	2008	2003	2008	2003	2008	2003	2008	2003	2008	2003	2008
Lowest	17.0	22.1	2.4	1.4	79.6	75.7	0.3	0.2	0.7	0.6	941	744
Second	24.1	41.7	6.0	7.0	69.0	50.2	0.6	1.0	0.4	0.1	809	641
Third	32.8	53.5	7.9	8.6	58.5	36.5	0.2	0.7	0.7	0.7	721	549
Fourth	57.3	68.8	15.5	11.3	26.4	19.6	0.6	0.0	0.2	1.0	617	560
Highest	68.0	71.5	21.4	21.2	9.2	6.6	0.0	0.3	1.4	0.3	551	415
Total	36.3	48.4	9.4	8.7	53.4	42.0	0.6	0.5	0.6	0.5	3,639	2,909

Source: GSS, GHS, and ICF Macro 2009.
Note: Figures pertain to women who gave birth in previous five years.

Table 2.6 Percent of Pregnant Women in Ghana Who Sought Assistance During Delivery, 2003 and 2008

Wealth quintile	Doctor		Nurse/midwife/ auxiliary midwife		Traditional birth attendant		Relative/other		No one		Don't know		Number of births	
	2003	2008	2003	2008	2003	2008	2003	2008	2003	2008	2003	2008	2003	2008
Lowest	1.6	2.2	19.0	24.2	37.8	49.8	37.5	15.0	3.3	4.2	0.8	0.7	941	744
Second	3.0	5.8	28.9	47.9	44.3	30.5	21.1	12.1	2.4	3.4	0.4	0.4	809	641
Third	3.4	9.2	39.9	58.9	37.2	22.1	16.7	6.3	2.0	2.0	0.8	0.7	721	549
Fourth	10.5	17.6	62.6	66.4	19.2	11.0	5.9	1.7	1.7	1.6	0.2	0.3	617	560
Highest	20.2	28.6	70.2	66.9	4.7	3.6	2.9	0.6	0.6	0.3	1.4	0.3	551	415
Total	6.6	11.0	40.5	48.6	31.0	27.7	19.1	8.1	2.2	2.5	0.7	0.5	3,639	2,909

Source: Author, based on data from GSS, GHS, and ICF Macro 2009.
Note: Figures pertain to women who gave birth in previous five years.

Table 2.7 Percent of Pregnant Women in Ghana Who Sought Assistance During Delivery, by Wealth Quintile and Insurance Status, 2008

Wealth quintile	Doctor		Nurse		Auxiliary midwife		Community health worker		Trained traditional birth attendant		Untrained traditional birth attendant	
	Insured	Uninsured	Insured	Uninsured	Insured	Uninsured	Insured	Uninsured	Insured	Uninsured	Insured	Uninsured
Lowest	7.0	1.2	40.8	24.0	1.7	1.1	6.9	0.6	11.3	22.7	43.3	49.3
Second	3.5	7.9	57.3	33.7	17.6	4.8	6.8	3.3	17.5	28.7	24.0	14.5
Middle	12.3	11.6	81.0	52.7	8.0	5.1	0	1.1	15.3	24.5	12.0	17.8
Fourth	18.3	13.3	81.0	79.3	7.8	6.3	0	0	7.9	18.6	3.8	0
Highest	27.8	36.5	86.7	88.1	12.6	3.2	0	2.4	0	0	2.9	3.1
Total	15.5	9.8	73.0	45.8	9.7	3.8	2.0	1.5	9.4	22.0	13.6	22.9

Source: Authors' calculation, based on data from GSS, GHS, and ICF Macro 2009.

Note: Figures pertain to women who gave birth in previous year.

Table 2.8 Percent of Pregnant Women in Ghana Who Delivered in a Health Facility, by Wealth Quintile and Insurance Status, 2008

Wealth quintile	Government hospital		Health center		Private hospital[a]		Other[b]		Home	
	Insured	Uninsured	Insured	Uninsured	Insured	Uninsured	Insured	Uninsured	Insured	Uninsured
Lowest	32.0	11.4	23.9	12.3	0	0	1.6	2.6	65.2	87.8
Second	37.9	21.4	33.0	15.8	3.7	5.5	7.4	6.8	43.2	64.8
Middle	56.9	35.0	21.7	17.5	7.5	6.3	6.2	7.5	28.0	50.2
Fourth	74.0	54.5	16.3	13.7	8.7	7.1	3.7	7.9	13.0	28.4
Highest	65.7	71.8	9.5	9.6	16.1	20.7	9.4	0	5.1	4.7
Total	57.6	30.2	19.4	14.1	8.2	5.5	5.8	5.2	25.7	58.6

Source: Authors' calculation, based on data from GSS, GHS, and ICF Macro 2009.

Note: Figures pertain to women who gave birth in previous year.

a. Private hospital clinic, Family Planning/Planned Parenthood Association of Ghana, clinic, maternity home, or other private facility.

b. Facilities other than home or facilities owned by public or private medical sector. Detailed responses were not provided in the micro data.

Figure 2.1   Average Month of Pregnancy During First Prenatal Visit by Women in Ghana, by Wealth Quintile and Insurance Status, 2008

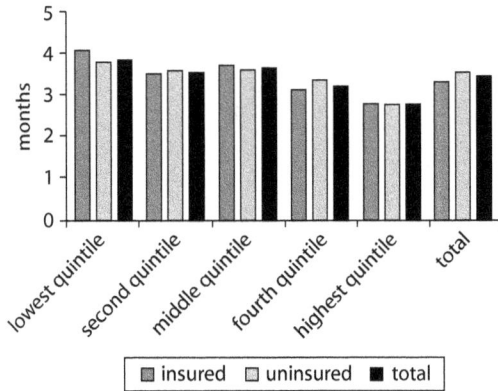

Source: Authors' calculation, based on data from GSS, GHS, and ICF Macro 2009.
Note: Figures pertain to women who gave birth in previous year.

of their total expenditures on health care in 2005/06—more than six times the 0.5 percent spent by the top four quintiles (figure 2.2).

Table 2.9 shows the share of household health spending as a percentage of total household expenditure for various thresholds. Only 1.4 percent of households in Ghana spent 10 percent or more of their total expenditures on health care. This figure is very low compared with some other countries (in Bangladesh and Vietnam, for example, 15 percent of households are above this threshold, according to Van Doorslaer and others 2007). These households are concentrated in the lowest quintile.

Figure 2.3 ranks households by per capita consumption expenditure (x-axis) and per capita expenditure on health (y-axis). The spikes show the difference between expenditure of the household before and after health spending. For households near the poverty line, incurring health expenditures can push them into poverty.

The poverty headcount (the first line in table 2.10) indicates the percent of households falling below the poverty line. Two official poverty lines are used in the analysis: the lower poverty line of GH¢288 per person per year and the higher poverty line of GH¢371.[1] In 2005/06, 31.8 percent of the population fell below the lower poverty line; excluding out-of-pocket health spending raised this figure to 32.0 percent. This means that 0.2 percent of the population was not counted as poor using conventional poverty measures. Out-of-pocket spending raised the average shortfall from the poverty line by GH¢0.3, a percent change of almost 1 percent. Among the poor, this gap increased by GH¢0.1, a 0.3 percent percentage

Figure 2.2   Share of Spending Devoted to Health Care in Ghana, by Consumption Quintile, 2005/06

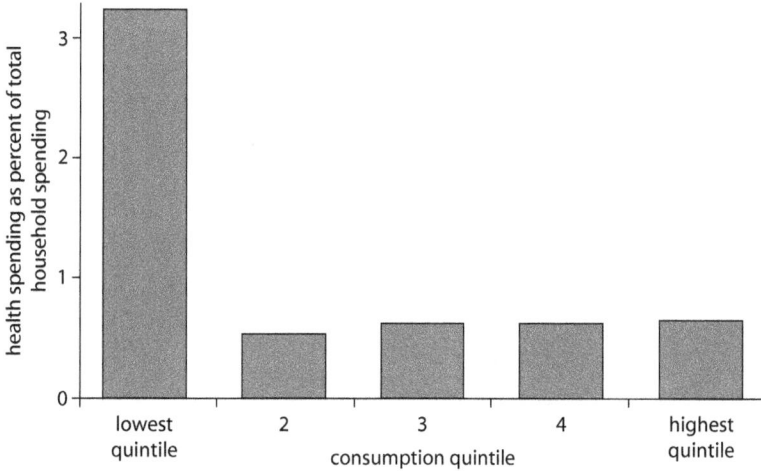

Source: Authors' calculation, based on data from GSS 2008.

Table 2.9   Catastrophic Expenditure Headcounts in Ghana, by Threshold, 2005/06

Consumption quintile	Percent of total household spending allocated to health care				
	5	10	15	25	40
Lowest	4.3	3.3	2.9	2.9	2.9
Second	1.8	0.6	0.3	0.0	0.0
Middle	2.5	1.1	0.4	0.0	0.0
Fourth	2.3	1.0	0.4	0.1	0.0
Highest	2.3	1.1	0.6	0.2	0.1
Total	2.7	1.4	0.9	0.6	0.6

Source: Authors' calculation, based on data from GSS 2008.

change. These figures imply that more households originally classified as nonpoor were reclassified as poor as a result of out-of-pocket payments than there were poor people who were pushed into deeper poverty because of health payments. The same trend is observed for the upper poverty line.

Benefit and Financing Incidence
Assessing the benefit and financing incidence of Ghana's health system is problematic, because of the lack of recent household-level consumption

Figure 2.3   Per Capita Household Expenditure in Ghana, Gross and Net of Health Spending, 2005/06

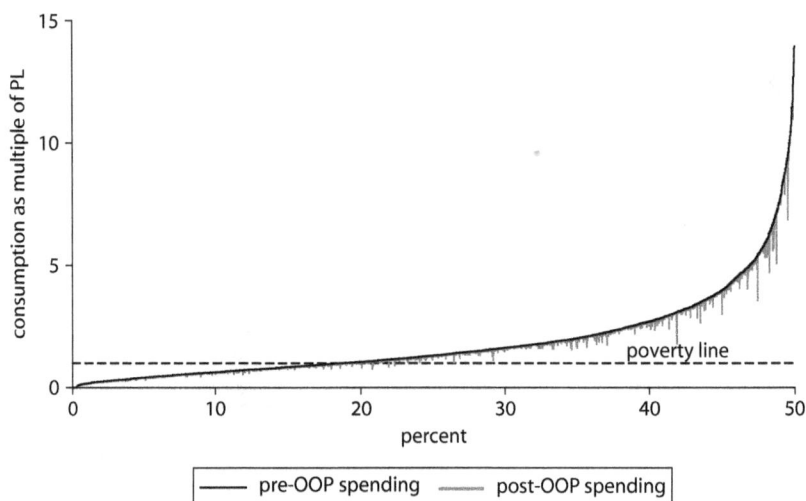

Source: Authors' calculation, based on data from GSS 2008.
Note: OOP = out of pocket; PL = poverty line.

Table 2.10   Poverty Rates in Ghana Before and After Out-of-Pocket Health Expenditures, 2005/2006
(cedis)

Poverty line/indicator	Expenditure, including out-of-pocket expenses	Expenditure, excluding out-of-pocket expenses	Change	Percentage change
Lower poverty line (GH¢288/year)				
Percent in poverty	31.8	32.0	0.2	0.6
Average shortfall from poverty line	33.4	33.7	0.3	0.9
Average shortfall from poverty line among the poor	36.4	36.5	0.1	0.3
Upper poverty line *(GH¢371/year)*				
Percent in poverty	44.5	44.8	0.3	0.7
Average shortfall from the poverty line	64.9	65.4	0.5	0.8
Average shortfall from the poverty line among the poor	39.3	39.4	0.1	0.3

Source: Authors' calculation, based on data from GSS 2008.

and expenditure data. There is a clear need for another Ghana Living Standards Survey–type study in 2012/2013 in order to monitor the impacts of Ghana's overall health financing arrangements and the NHIS on the critical health systems goals of equity and financial protection.

Based on the most recent data (from 2005/2006), a World Bank report on health equity and financial protection in Ghana (World Bank 2012) finds that government subsidies for inpatient and outpatient hospital care are pro-rich and subsidies for health centers and health posts are pro-poor. As health centers and health posts account for less than 17 percent of total health spending, total subsidies on health tend to favor the better-off.

Using 2006 household data augmented by a special 2008 SHIELD household survey, Akazili and others (2011) assess the benefit incidence of both the overall health financing system and the NHIS.[2] They find that Ghana's various tax levies are progressive but that out-of-pocket spending and NHIS voluntary enrollee premiums tend to be regressive. Overall, they find the financing of both the overall health system and the NHIS to be generally progressive (Akazili and others 2011).[3]

These analyses suggest that the financing incidence of Ghana's health system appears to be generally progressive but that the benefit incidence of Ghana's health financing system could be improved. Improvements in benefit incidence would result from better targeting, given the pro-rich eligibility bias of the NHIS, some of which may be attributable to the stringent definition of indigent and the need for better outreach. Although the premium schedule for informal sector enrollees is related to income, in practice most individuals wind up paying the same minimal premium, as a result of a lack of good instruments for means testing (Hendriks 2010). Better means testing would improve the progressivity of these premiums.

The still significant out-of-pocket spending, which accounted for 37 percent of total health spending in 2009, is the major factor contributing to regressive financing. As the NHIS expands to the rest of the population, in principle financed by largely progressive revenue sources, the progressivity of the financing system should improve, everything else equal.

Consumer Responsiveness

The third dimension of health system performance is consumer responsiveness. A properly functioning health system should respond efficiently and effectively to consumers. A responsive system ensures that client expectations are met, complaints are addressed, and quality of care is not compromised. Consumer satisfaction and responsiveness may also affect service utilization. Introduction of the NHIS has raised concerns that increased utilization of services may compromise the quality of care.

The National Development Planning Commission's report on the 2008 Citizens' Assessment Survey of the NHIS included citizens' feedback on the benefit package, the quality of service, and the affordability of health care. Overall, the scheme's performance was rated as high: about 92 percent of insured members reported being either "very satisfied" or "satisfied" with the scheme. Dissatisfaction levels were low: less than 7 percent of the insured and less than 11 percent of the partially insured reported being "dissatisfied" with the performance of the scheme.

This pattern of satisfaction is consistent across socioeconomic groups and regions. About 75 percent of the top income quintile and 82 percent of the bottom quintile reported being "satisfied" or "very satisfied" with the scheme's performance. In every region except Greater Accra, more than 76 percent of respondents reported being "very satisfied" or "satisfied." Respondents who were "satisfied" with the scheme were most satisfied by the publicity or educational campaign of the scheme. Respondents who were not registered with the scheme indicated that premium collection and utilization of resources were areas of concern.

The survey also asked respondents to compare their experiences of the health system before and after the introduction of the NHIS (figure 2.4). The most important benefit cited was the low cost of treatment. Seventy percent of respondents revealed that as a result of the scheme they are now able to access medical care at an affordable cost. The Western Region was the only exception to this finding. About 40–45 percent of respondents revealed that the availability of nurses and drugs, the cleanliness of facilities, and treatment of patients by staff had improved.

Feedback from consumers on the overall quality of health care delivery is available through the Core Welfare Indicators Questionnaire (CWIQ) survey published by the Ghana Statistical Service. The survey provides a picture of poverty and living conditions at the national, regional, and district levels. It has been conducted twice, in 1997 and in 2003. Given that the latest version is almost 10 years old, its relevance for capturing current consumer sentiments may be diminished. Nonetheless, under the health section, it collects information on client satisfaction with the health system. A comparison of the consumer satisfaction indicators for the two years suggests that client satisfaction increased. In 1997, 57 percent of people who used health services were satisfied with the

Figure 2.4 Consumer Satisfaction with Ghana's National Health Insurance System, 2008

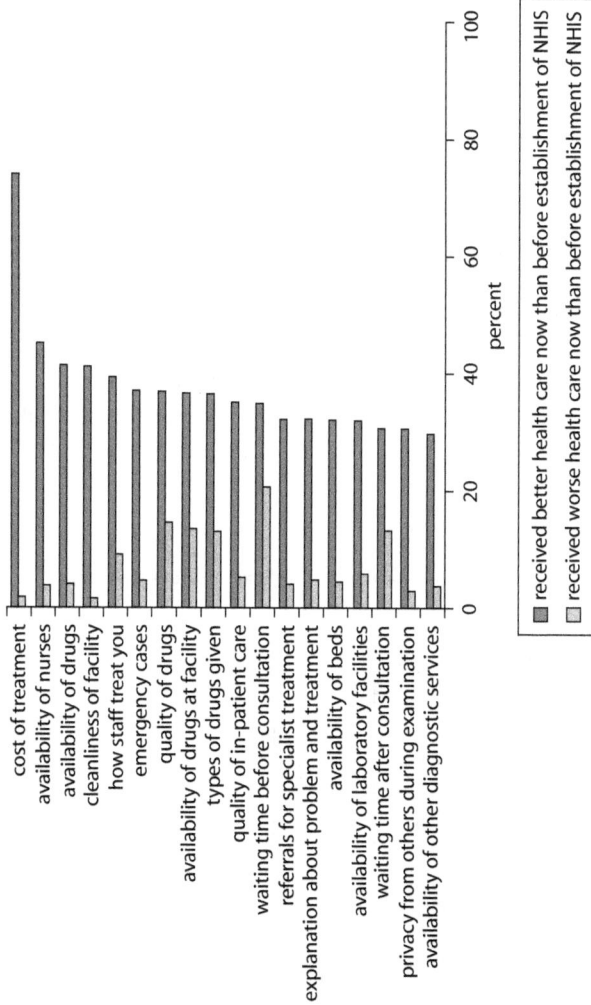

Source: NDPC 2009.

services they received, whereas in 2003 this figure rose to 79 percent. Regionally, the Central Region had the highest level of satisfied consumers (67 percent) in 1997, while the Ashanti Region had the highest (86 percent) in 2003. There is little variation in level of satisfaction across income groups (figure 2.5).

A 2006 review of six research projects (cited in the 2007–11 Strategic Plan of the Quality Assurance Department in the Institutional Care Division of the Ghana Health Service) commissioned by the Health Research Unit of the Ghana Health Service indicated that users of health services were "very satisfied" with specific programs and services but were "dissatisfied" with long wait times, poor personnel attitudes, illegal charges, and unclean environments. These findings are corroborated by a study by Turkson (2009), which reports that 89 percent of respondents were "very satisfied"'or "satisfied" with the service they received during their visit to various facilities.[4] Some participants in the study noted that insufficient and rude staff, long wait times, and transportation limitations reduced their satisfaction with the care they received.

Variations in the quality of care at different facilities also reduced consumer satisfaction. In the Lawra, Dangme West, and Ejisu-Juaben

Figure 2.5   Consumer Satisfaction with Medical Services in Ghana

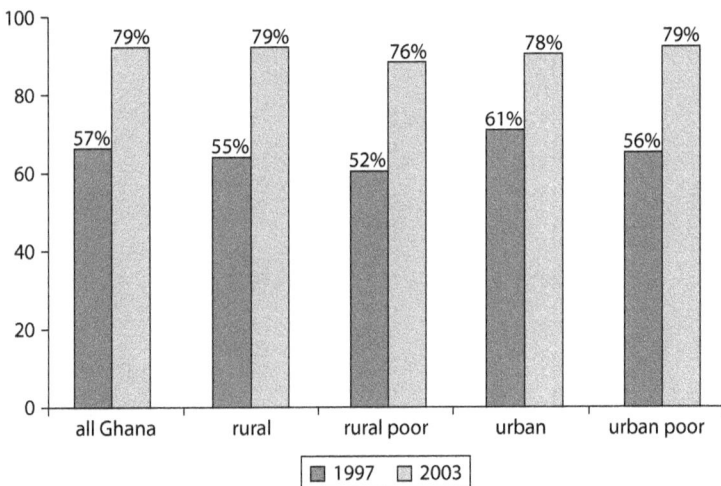

Source: GSS 1997, 2003.
Note: Health satisfaction is defined for people who consulted a health practitioner in the four weeks preceding the survey and who cited no problems.

districts, 63 percent of users surveyed reported being satisfied with the health delivery system (Nketsiah-Amponsah (2009). Users of private medical care reported higher levels of satisfaction than respondents who obtained services from other providers, even after controlling for socio-economic and demographic factors.[5] Dissatisfaction was highest with pharmacists and sellers of over-the-counter drugs. Consumers of private medical care increased their satisfaction levels by 31 percentage points, significantly more than users of public facilities, whose satisfaction was increased by only 19 percentage points. Provider characteristics such as distance to users and long wait times were correlated with sources of dissatisfaction.

Both studies acknowledge the limitations of measuring consumer satisfaction, which is subjective and can be influenced by such factors as previous experiences, physical and psychological health, and personal and societal values. Moreover, findings based on a purposive sample may not necessarily reflect the sentiments of the larger population.

These caveats notwithstanding, most consumers of health care in Ghana seem to be "satisfied" with the service they receive, although they complain about long wait times and the negative attitudes of some health workers. The high proportion of satisfied consumers is surprising giving the many challenges associated with accessing health care. But as Nketsiah-Amponsah (2009) notes, "satisfaction" may be an indication that in resource-constrained environments with limited alternatives, consumers of health care simply become content with the status quo.

Annex 2A. Performance Assessment of Ghana's Health System

This annex analyzes the performance of Ghana's system in two ways. First, it assesses changes in health outcomes (under-five mortality, maternal mortality, and life expectancy); delivery system inputs (number of beds, number of physicians) for 1960–2009; and total, public, and private health spending in Ghana and African comparators over the 1995–2009 period. Second, it benchmarks Ghana's performance for the latest year available (generally 2009) against other countries in the world with similar levels of income and spending on health (for outcomes and inputs only).

Health Outcome, Input, and Expenditure Trends over Time
This section examines various measures of health outcomes, inputs, and spending in Ghana and African comparators over time.

Outcomes. Under-five mortality in Ghana fell between 1960 and 2009 (figure 2A.1). Ghana started from a much lower base than most of its neighboring countries and has made limited progress in reducing this rate. As a result, Ghana, like many other countries in Sub-Saharan Africa, is not on track to meet the MDG target of reducing under-five mortality by two-thirds between 1990 and 2015, according to the United Nations Development Programme (UNDP 2010). A recent report, however, suggests that if Ghana augments its recently expanded efforts, it might be able to reach the target (Nakamura and others 2011).

A similar picture emerges for maternal mortality. Ghana started with a lower base level, but like many of its neighbors, the rate has fallen too slowly for it to meet the MDG target of reducing maternal mortality by three-quarters between 1990 and 2015 (figure 2A.2).

Life expectancy in Ghana started from a much higher base than most of its neighbors and has risen steadily since 1960. At 63.4 years in 2009, it is higher than all of its African comparator countries except Tunisia (figure 2A.3).

Figure 2A.1   Under-Five Mortality Rate in Ghana and Selected African Comparators, 1960–2009

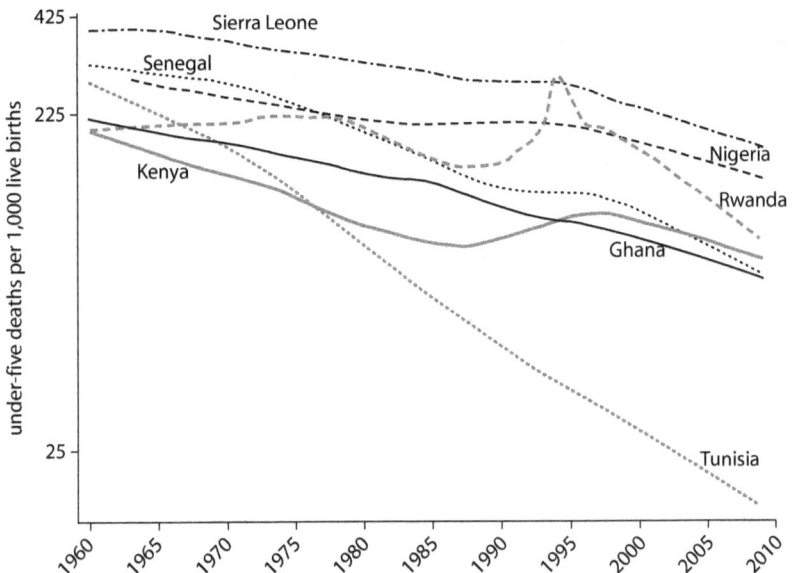

Source: World Bank 2011b.
Note: y-axis is log scale.

Figure 2A.2   Maternal Mortality Ratio in Ghana and Selected African Comparators, 1990–2008

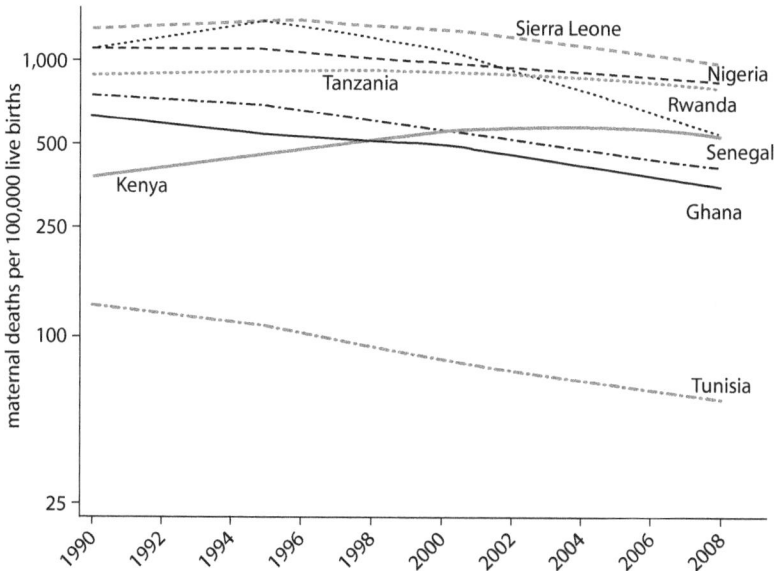

Source: World Bank 2011b.
Note: y-axis is log scale.

Inputs. The number of physicians and hospitals beds per capita was close to the median of Ghana's African comparators in both 1960 and 2009.[6] Although the number of physicians per capita increased significantly over the period (increasing rapidly between 1990 and 2005 but declining thereafter), the number of hospital beds per capita has been declining since 1985 (figures 2A.4 and 2A.5).

Expenditure. Figure 2A.6 compares trends in total, public, private, and out-of-pocket health spending in local currency units, adjusting for population growth and inflation. Absolute and per capita levels of total health spending in nominal and constant (that is, real) terms increased over this period, with the largest increases in public spending.

Table 2A.1 displays the nominal elasticities of total, private, and public health spending with respect to GDP for 1995–2009 as well as for the 1995–2003 and 2004–09 subperiods. Over the entire 1995–2009 period, annual nominal health spending in Ghana increased almost 3 percentage points faster than GDP (elasticity of 1.028). In contrast, average health

Figure 2A.3   Life Expectancy at Birth in Ghana and Selected African Comparators, 1960–2009

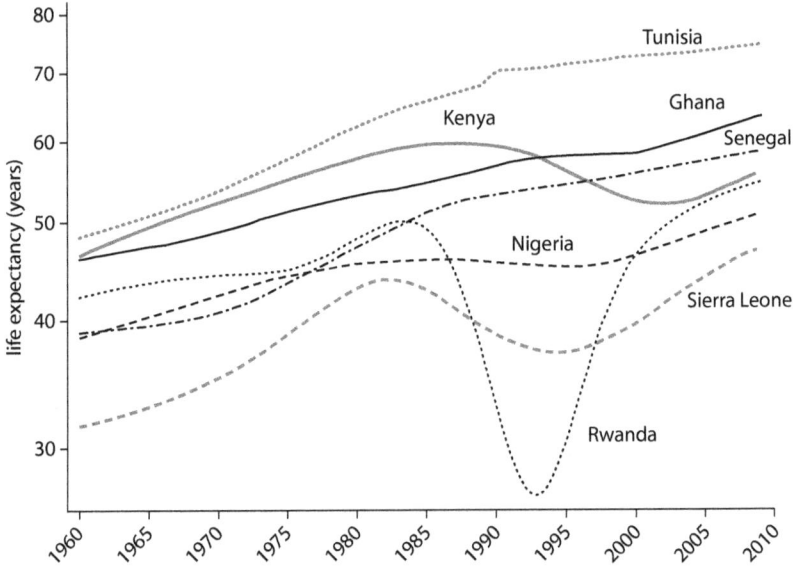

Source: World Bank 2011b.
Note: y-axis is log scale.

spending in Sub-Saharan African countries increased about 9 percent more rapidly than GDP (1.086). Annual public spending in Ghana increased about 13 percentage points more rapidly than GDP (1.130); private spending increased about 7 percentage points less rapidly (0.927). These figures compare with elasticities of 1.172 for public spending and 1.018 for private spending for Sub-Saharan Africa as a whole. For the 2004–09 (NHIS implementation) period, annual total health spending in Ghana increased at the same rate as GDP (1.000), public health spending increased 11 percentage points more rapidly (1.113), and private spending increased 13 percentage points less rapidly (0.872).

Table 2A.2 displays the nominal elasticities of total and public health spending in Ghana with respect to total government revenue and expenditures for 1995–2009 as well as for the 1995–2003 and 2004–09 subperiods. Over the 1995–2009 period, total health spending increased annually almost 8 percentage points less rapidly than total government revenue (elasticity of 0.921) and 1 percentage point more rapidly than total government spending (elasticity of 1.012). Over the same time period, annual

Figure 2A.4   Number of Physicians per 1,000 People in Ghana and Selected African Comparators, 1960–2009

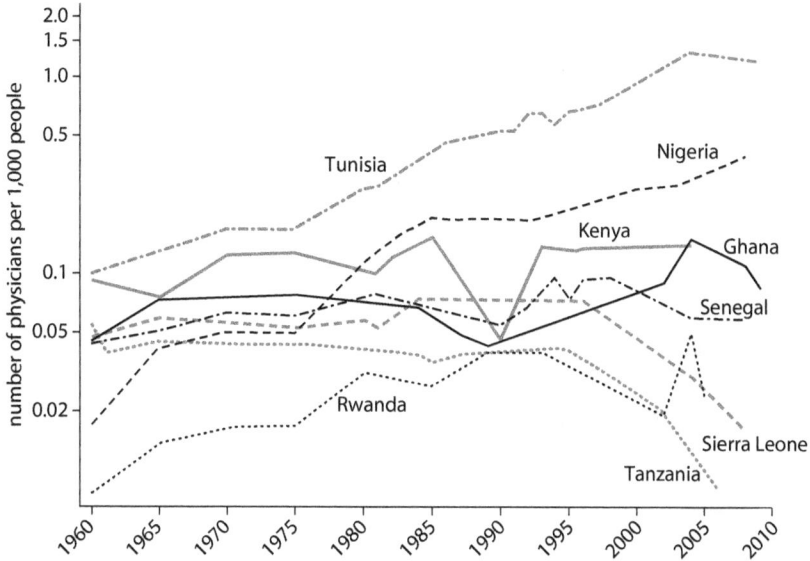

Source: World Bank 2011b.
Note: y-axis is log scale.

public health spending increased about 1 percentage point more rapidly than total government revenue (elasticity of 1.013) and 12 percentage points more rapidly than total government expenditure (elasticity of 1.119). For the 2004–09 (NHIS implementation period), total annual health spending increased about 3 percentage points more rapidly than total government revenue (elasticity of 1.030) and 9 percentage points less rapidly than total government spending (elasticity of 0.905). Annual public health spending increased about 15 percentage points more rapidly than total government revenue (elasticity of 1.148) and 2 percentage points more rapidly than expenditure (elasticity of 1.021).

Figure 2A.7 shows changes in the public, private, out-of-pocket, and externally funded shares of total health spending in Ghana. Although the share of external funding dropped from about 30 percent of total spending in the early 2000s to about 14 percent in 2009, the public share rose after 2004, except for a slight decrease in 2008 and 2009, which may have been related to the global financial crisis. The private

Figure 2A.5   Number of Hospital Beds per 1,000 People in Ghana and Selected African Comparators, 1960–2009

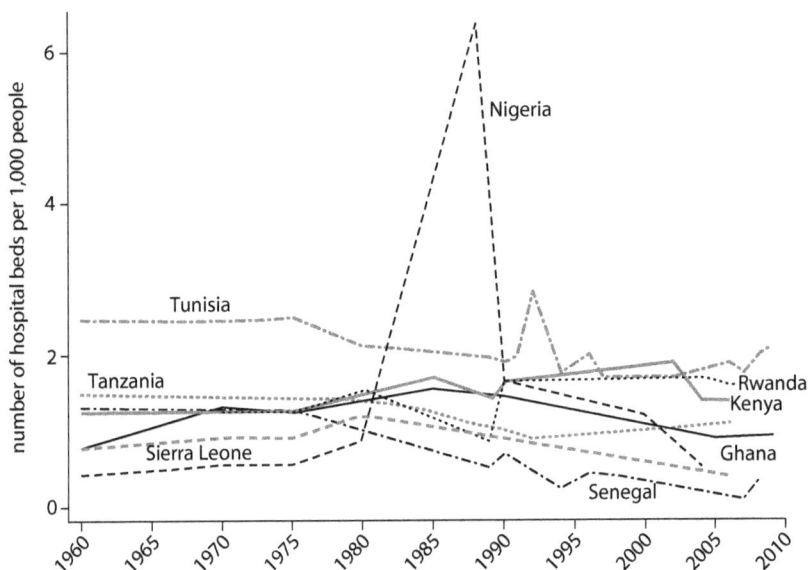

Source: World Bank 2011b.

and out-of-pocket shares declined except for a slight increase in 2008 and 2009. Thus, it would appear that the implementation of the NHIS in 2005 is associated with a larger share of public financing on health and a smaller share of out-of-pocket spending.

Ghana's out-of-pocket share declined from about 44 percent of total health spending in 1995 to 37 percent in 2009 (figure 2A.8).

One can also evaluate health spending in a single numeraire currency, such as the U.S. dollar, which facilitates absolute spending level comparisons with other countries. Figure 2A.9 shows Ghana's per capita health spending in nominal and real terms, in U.S. and international dollars. The results parallel the local currency unit analysis, showing that per capita spending increased, except in 2008 and 2009.

Ghana's nominal per capita health spending mirrors that of its African comparators except Tunisia (figure 2A.10).

Figure 2A.11 shows trends in total, public, private and out-of-pocket health spending in Ghana as a share of GDP.

Total health spending as a share of GDP fell from 5.3 percent to 4.9 percent of GDP over the 1995–2009 period. Public spending on

Figure 2A.6   Total and Per Capita Health Spending in Ghana, 1995–2009

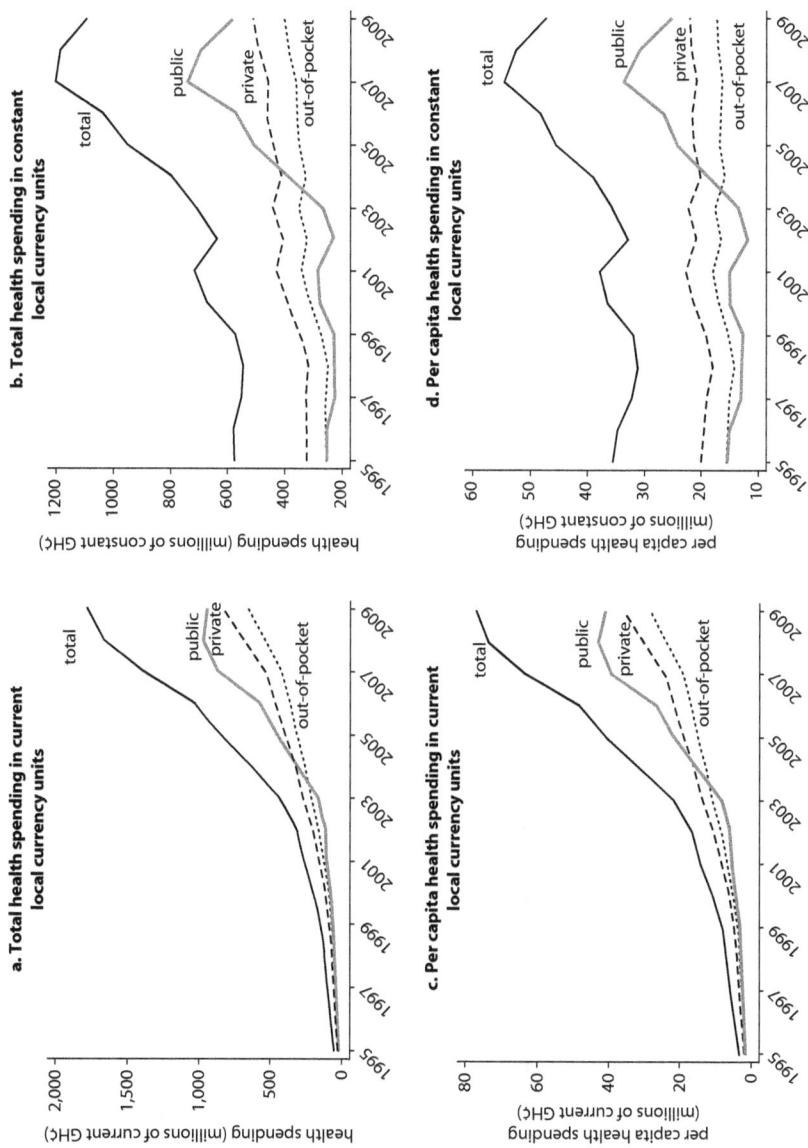

a. Total health spending in current
local currency units

b. Total health spending in constant
local currency units

c. Per capita health spending in current
local currency units

d. Per capita health spending in constant
local currency units

Source: WHO 2011.

61

Table 2A.1 Elasticity of Health Expenditure with Respect to GDP Growth in Ghana and Sub-Saharan Africa, 1995–2009

Entity	Total			Public			Private		
	1995–2009	1995–2003	2004–09	1995–2009	1995–2003	2004–09	1995–2009	1995–2003	2004–09
Ghana	1.028	0.935	1.000	1.130	0.862	1.113	0.927	0.983	0.872
Sub-Saharan Africa	1.086	—	—	1.172	—	—	1.018	—	—
Sub-Saharan Africa excluding South Africa	1.087	—	—	1.175	—	—	1.018	—	—

Source: WHO 2011.
Note: — Not available.

Table 2A.2   Elasticity of Total and Public Health Expenditure with Respect to Total Government Revenue and Expenditure in Ghana, 1995–2009

	Total health expenditure			Public health expenditure		
Item	1995–2009	1995–2003	2004–09	1995–2009	1995–2003	2004–09
Total government revenue	0.921	0.826	1.030	1.013	0.764	1.148
Total government spending	1.012	1.018	0.905	1.119	0.943	1.021

Source: WHO 2011.

Figure 2A.7   Composition of Total Health Spending in Ghana, 1995–2009

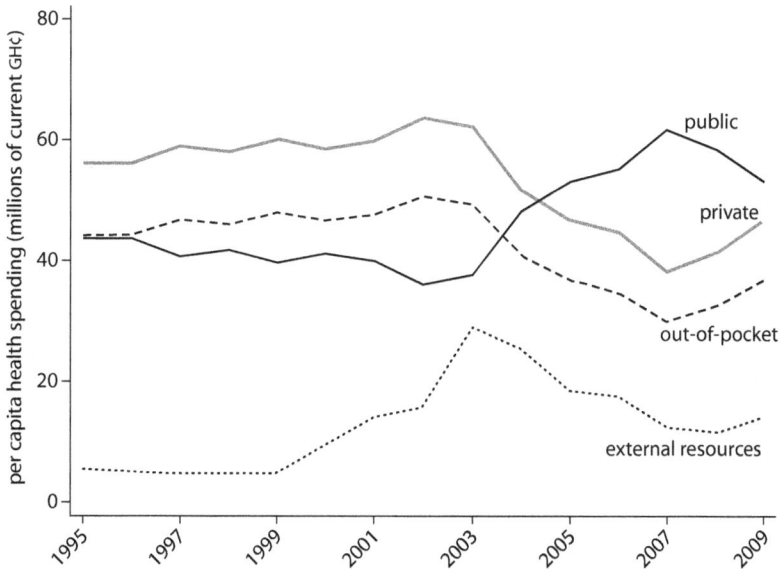

Source: WHO 2011.

health as a share of GDP increased significantly between 2004 and 2007, but its 2009 level was only slightly higher than its 1995 level. As a percentage of GDP, private and out-of-pocket spending declined steadily since 1995. Unlike its comparators, which increased the share of GDP they allocated to health, Ghana reduced the share of GDP it devoted to health (figure 2A.12). Its elasticity of health spending with respect to GDP (1.03) was lower than that of Sub-Saharan Africa as whole (elasticity of 1.09)

Figure 2A.8   Out-Of-Pocket Share of Health Spending in Ghana and Selected African Comparators, 1995–2009

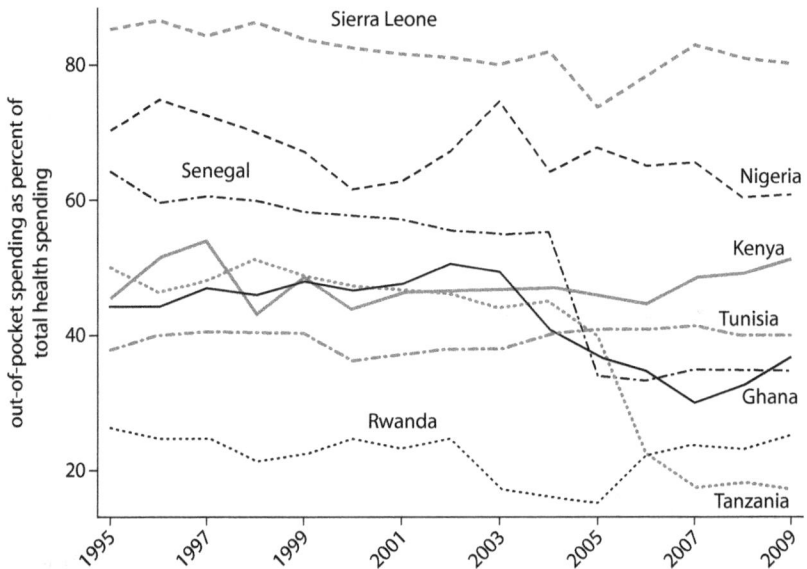

Source: WHO 2011.

Ghana's public spending on health as a share of GDP was only slightly higher than its 1995 level. It was lower than in several comparator countries (figure 2A.13) and lower than the Sub-Saharan Africa average (elasticity of 1.13 versus 1.17).

The share of the government budget devoted to health was higher in 2009 than in 1995. It was at about the level of comparators, with the exception of Rwanda and Tanzania, but below the 15 percent Abuja target (figure 2A.14). Government health spending in Ghana increased by about 12 percent a year more rapidly than overall government spending over 1995–2009 (see table 2A.2).

Benchmarking Ghana's Performance against Countries with Similar Levels of Income and Health Spending

Rigorous assessment of the performance of any health system is difficult for a number of well-known methodological and data reasons. For this reason, researchers often use global benchmarking of health outcomes, inputs, and health spending to provide an indication of how a country is performing relative to global averages for countries with comparable

Figure 2A.9   Per Capita Health Spending in Ghana, 1995–2009

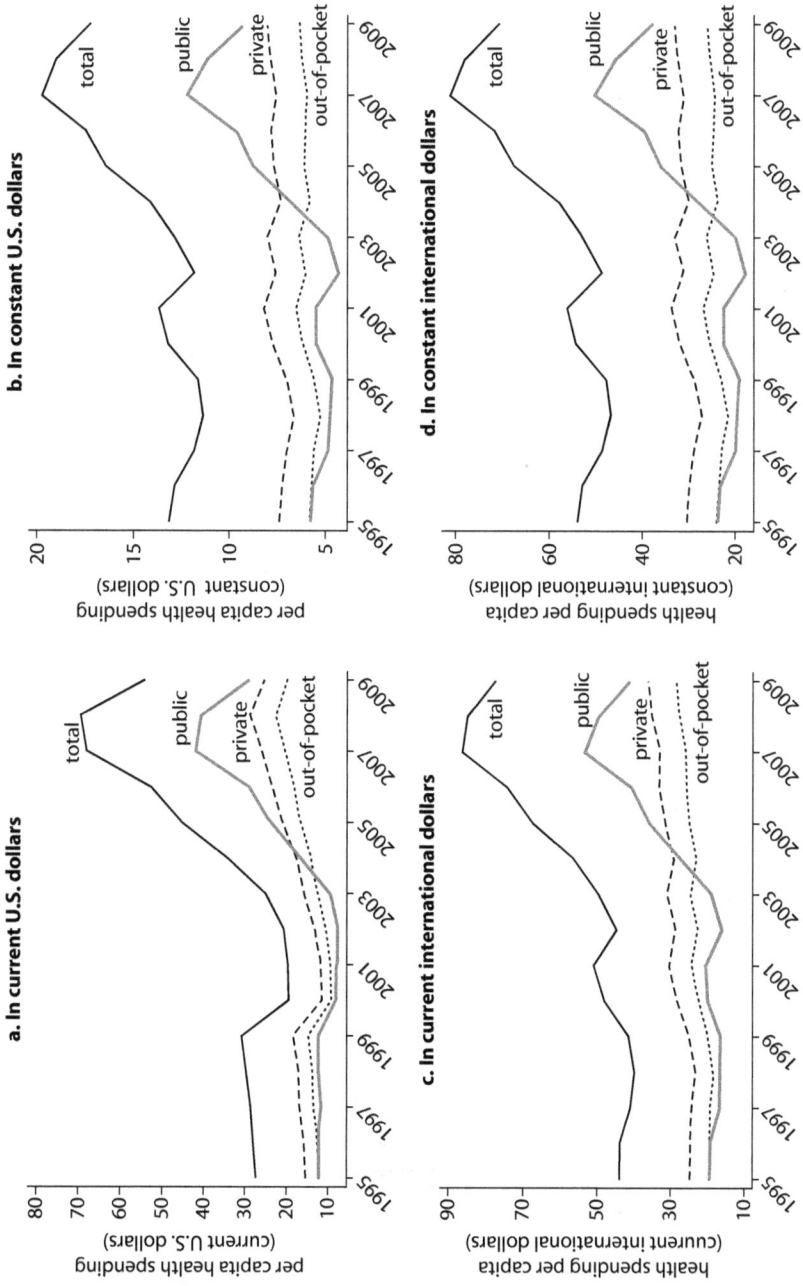

a. In current U.S. dollars

b. In constant U.S. dollars

c. In current international dollars

d. In constant international dollars

Source: WHO 2011.

Figure 2A.10   Nominal Per Capita Health Spending in Ghana and Selected African Comparators, 1995–2009

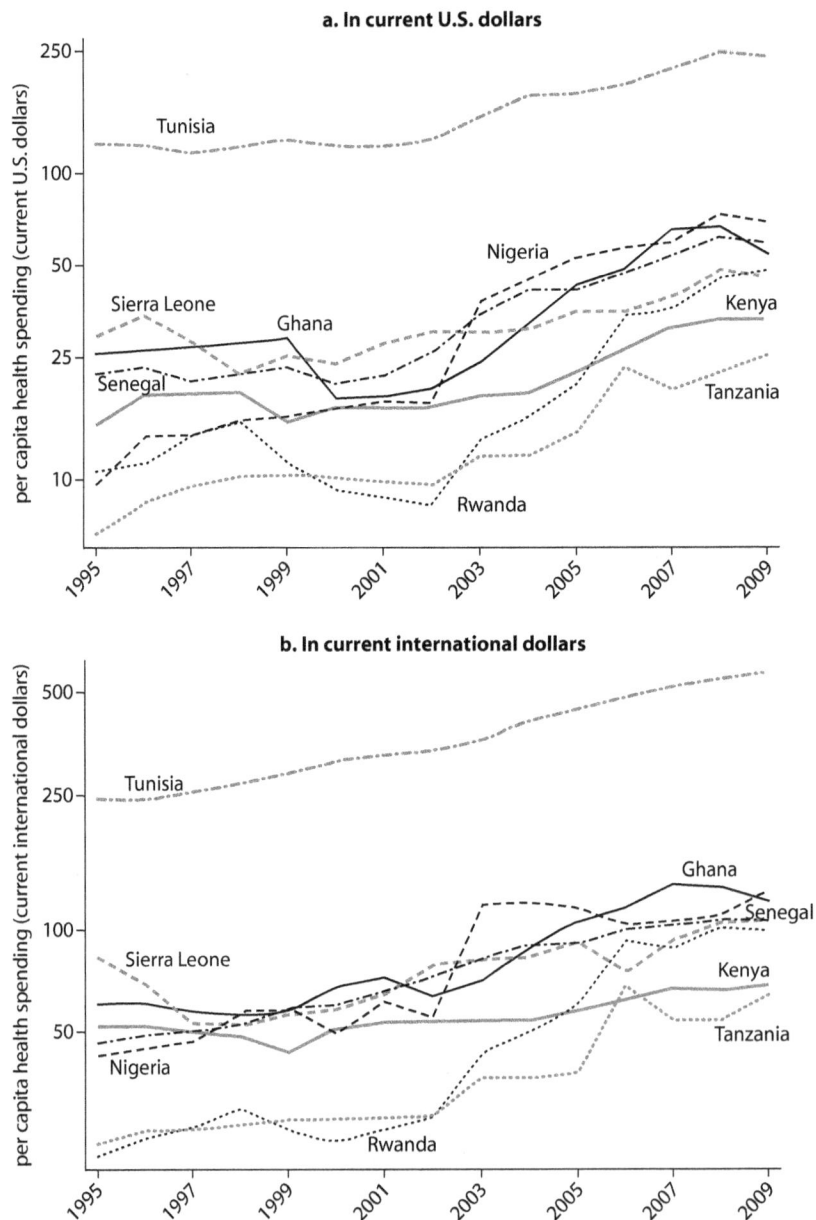

a. In current U.S. dollars

b. In current international dollars

Source: World Bank 2011.
Note: y-axis is log scale.

Figure 2A.11   Composition of Health Spending in Ghana as Percent of GDP, 1995–2009

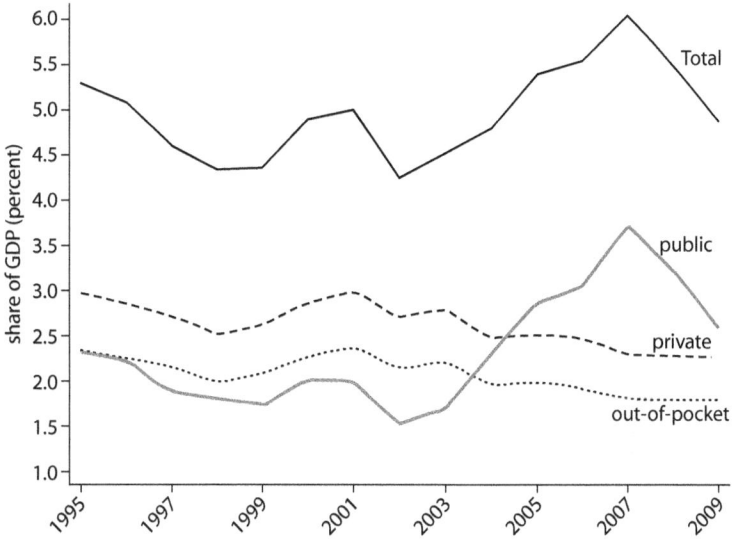

Source: WHO 2011.

Figure 2A.12   Total Spending on Health as Percent of GDP in Ghana and Selected African Comparators, 1995–2009

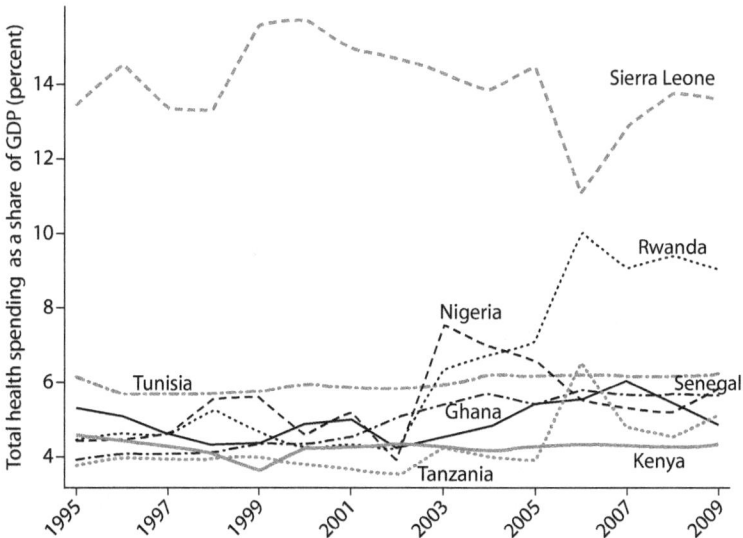

Source: WHO 2011.

Figure 2A.13   Public Spending on Health as Percent of GDP in Ghana and Selected African Comparators, 1995–2009

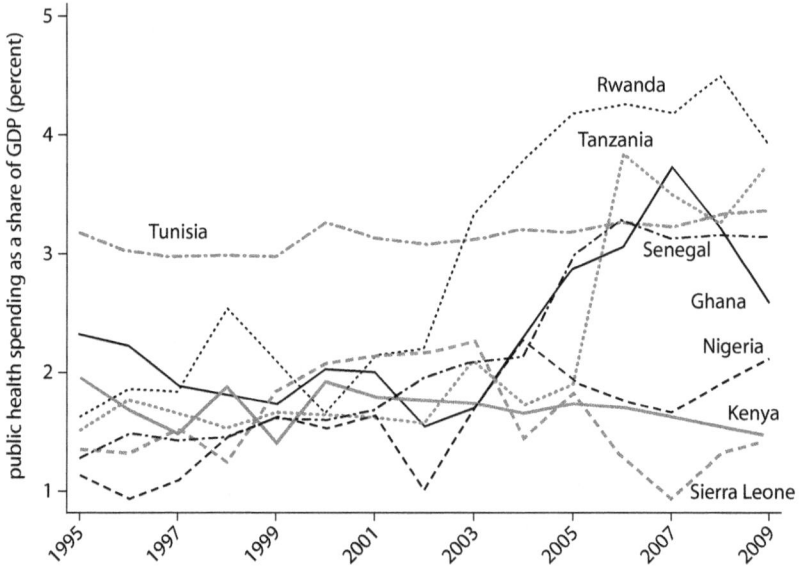

Source: WHO 2011.

Figure 2A.14   Public Spending on Health as Percent of Government Budget in Ghana and Selected African Comparators, 1995–2009

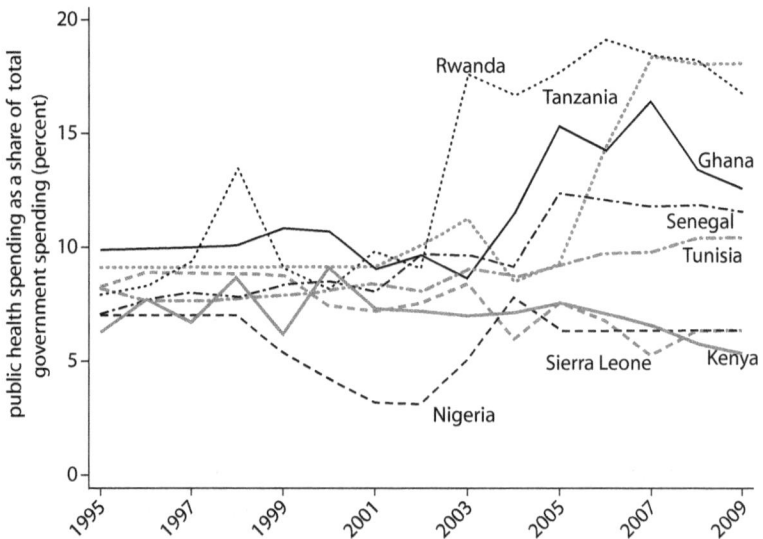

Source: WHO 2011.

income and health spending. Although there is nothing sacrosanct about a global average, it is one easy-to-measure metric for assessing comparative performance. Such assessments along a number of dimensions can provide useful information about sources of health spending, health outcomes, financial protection performance, and value for money. However, in interpreting these results, one must keep in mind that Ghana has only recently entered the ranks of lower-middle-income countries. Its institutions and health system's structures may not be strictly comparable to other countries that have held this status for a longer period of time.

Outcomes. Under-five mortality is higher in Ghana than in countries with comparable income and health spending (figure 2A.15).[7] The high rate of under-five mortality may partly reflect Ghana's only average adult female literacy level (figure 2A.16), the relatively low levels of skilled birth attendance (figure 2A.17), the lack of infrastructure and personnel in rural areas, and the excessive allocation of resources to tertiary care. Given that Ghana is not on track to achieve the MDG target for under-five mortality, it will be important to fully understand the factors responsible for Ghana's poor performance on this indicator, particularly now that Ghana is a lower-middle-income country.

Figure 2A.15   Under-Five Mortality in Ghana and Global Comparator Countries, 2009

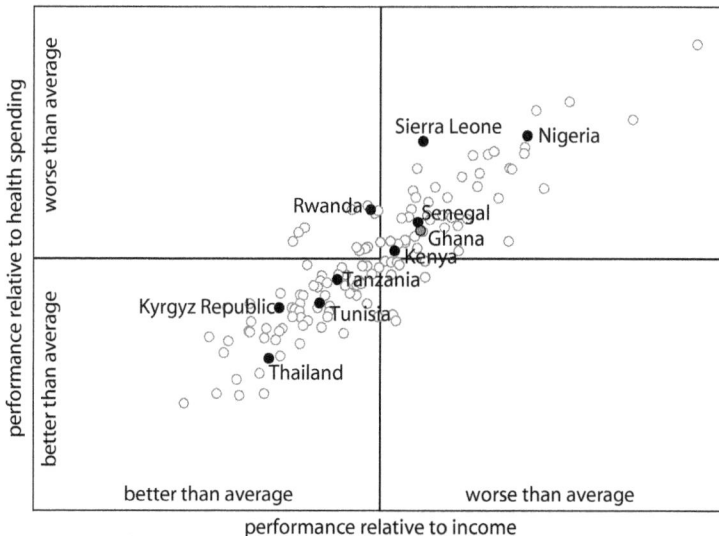

Sources: World Bank 2011b; WHO 2011.

Figure 2A.16   Women's Literacy in Ghana and Global Comparator Countries

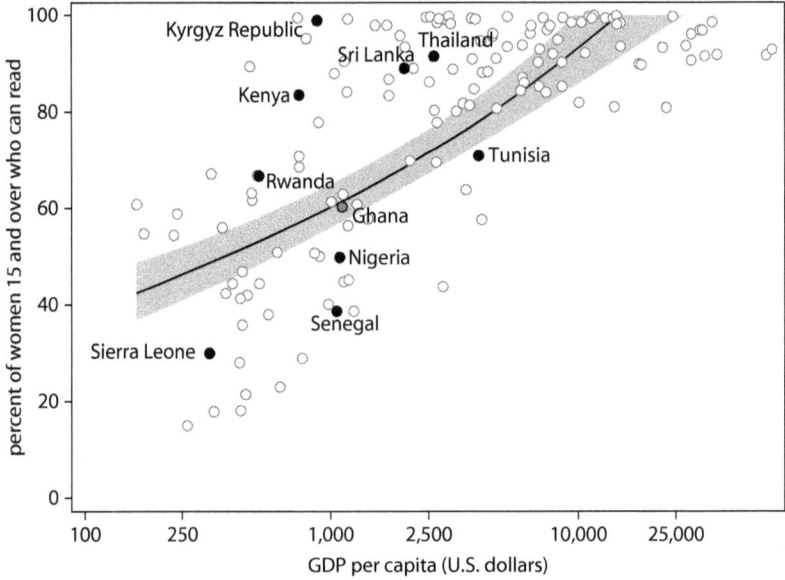

Sources: World Bank 2011b; WHO 2011.
Note: Both axes are log scale. Data are for latest year available.

Figure 2A.17   Birth Attendance by Skilled Health Workers in Ghana and Global Comparator Countries

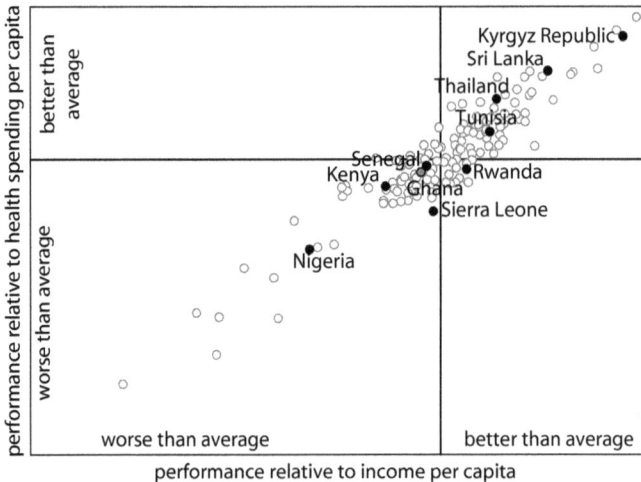

Sources: World Bank 2011b; WHO 2011.
Note: Both axes are log scale. Data are latest available between 2003 and 2008.

A similar picture emerges with respect to maternal mortality, which is much higher in Ghana than in global comparator countries (figure 2A.18). Recent changes to the NHIS that eliminate waiting periods for children and provide free care for pregnant women should lead to reductions in both under-five and maternal mortality.

Life expectancy in Ghana is higher than in its global comparators (figure 2A.19). It increased by almost three years between 2004 and 2009, rising to 63.4 years in 2009.

There is no single metric for measuring a country's overall health performance. But disability-adjusted life years (DALYs) are often used as an aggregate measure of overall health status, measuring how effectively countries extend life and limit disability. The most recent global data available for all countries are for 2004, before the NHIS was implemented. Nevertheless, it is useful to see how Ghana performed relative to global comparators on this aggregate health outcome measure.

In 2004, Ghana appears to have had more premature death and disability than its global comparators (figure 2A.20). Like the comparisons of Ghana with both African and global comparators, these figures suggest

Figure 2A.18   Maternal Mortality in Ghana and Global Comparator Countries

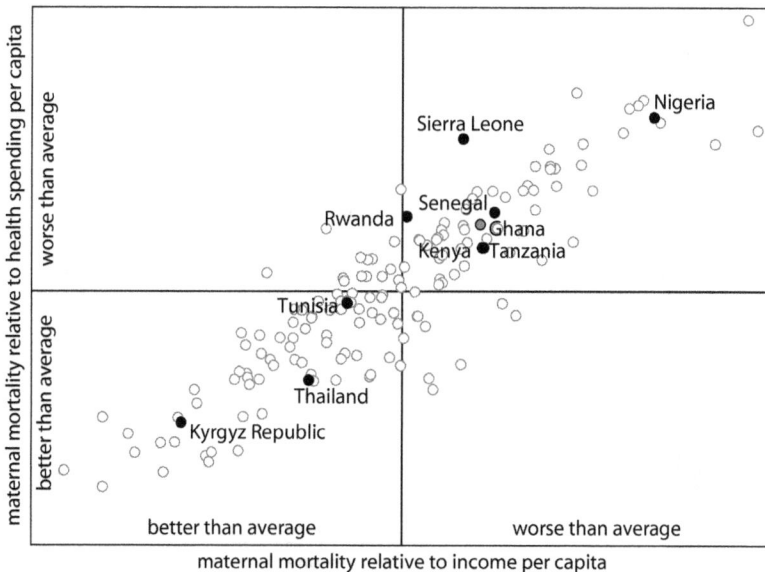

Sources: World Bank 2011b; WHO 2011.
Note: The latest data are for 2008.

Figure 2A.19   Life Expectancy in Ghana and Global Comparator Countries

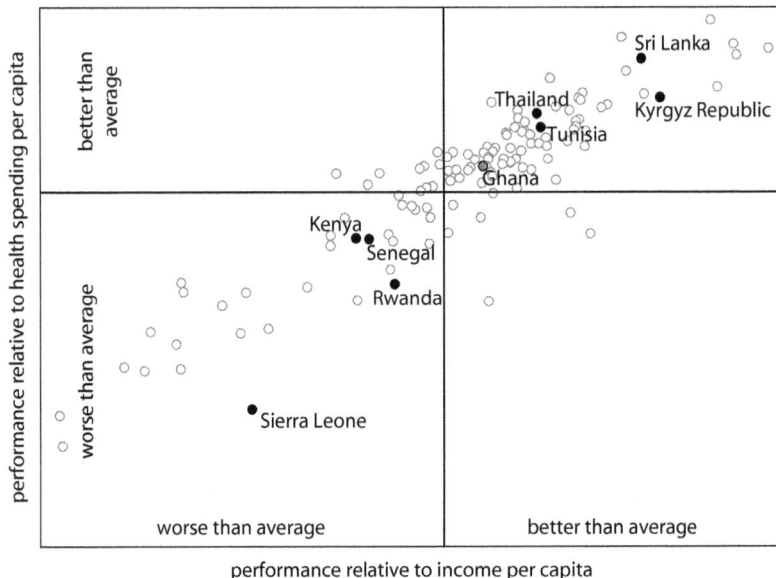

Sources: World Bank 2011b; WHO 2011.
Note: Both axes are log scale.

Figure 2A.20   Disability-Adjusted Life Years (DALYs) Per Capita in Ghana and Global Comparator Countries, 2004

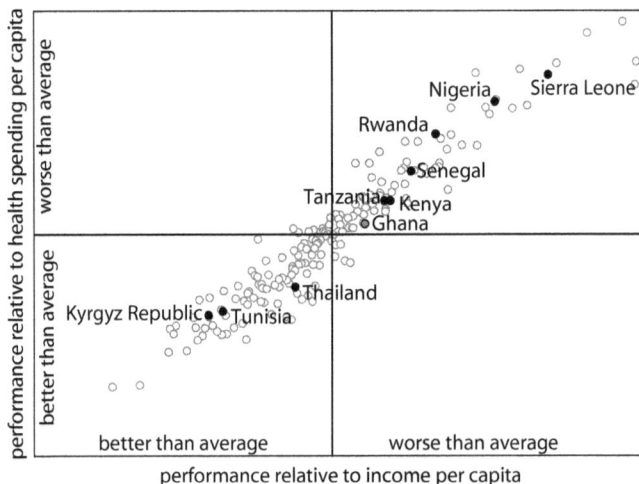

Sources: World Bank 2011b; WHO 2011.
Note: Both axes are log scale.

that Ghana's performance on some key health outcomes could be improved.

Many countries in Africa have weak health outcomes for their level of income and health spending. It is plausible that Ghana and Africa more generally face greater health risks, as a result of climate, malaria, HIV/AIDs, and other factors. Future analyses of this type should try to control for these underlying conditions.

Inputs. Ghana's hospital bed to population ratio is below the levels found in global comparators (figure 2A.21). The distribution (and staffing) of beds is also an important issue, given the large urban-rural disparities in Ghana.

The number of physicians in Ghana per 1,000 people is well below the number found in its global comparators (figure 2A.22). Of course, one must look beyond the total numbers of physicians and consider the specialty mix, relative remuneration, location, productivity, and numbers and mix of other health workers as well as equipment and facilities.

Figure 2A.21   Number of Hospital Beds per 1,000 People in Ghana and Global Comparator Countries

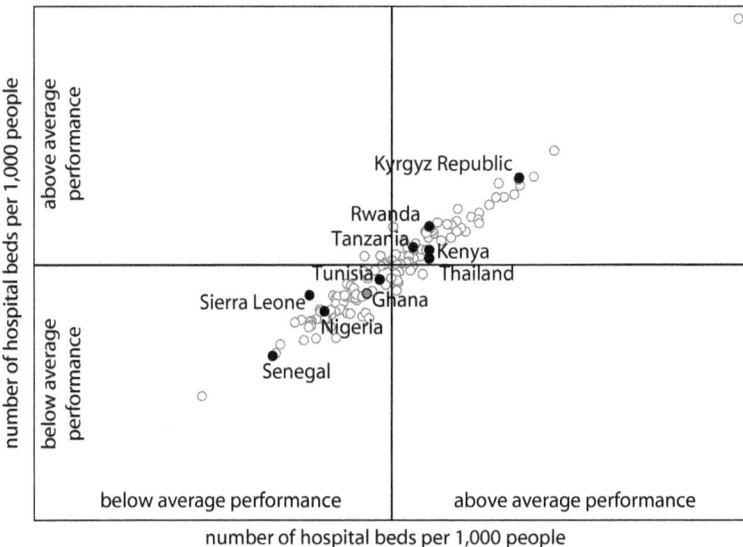

Sources: World Bank 2011b; WHO 2011.
Note: Data are for latest year available.

Figure 2A.22   Number of Physicians per 1,000 People in Ghana and Global Comparator Countries

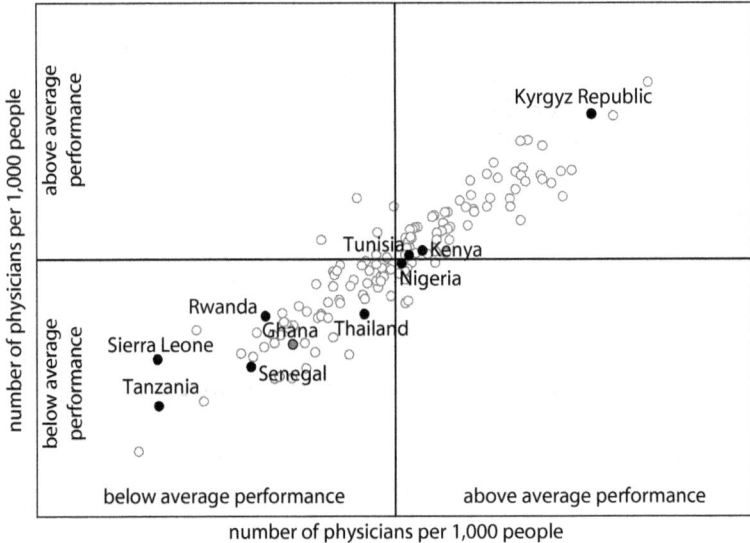

Sources: World Bank 2011b; WHO 2011.
Note: Data are for latest year available.

Ghana's level of total health workers per capita is low relative to its global comparators (figure 2A.23). Its relatively weak performance on health outcomes may be partially attributable to its relatively low ratios of doctors and other health workers and to the distribution and efficiency of its human and physical infrastructure.

The analysis suggests that relative to countries at similar levels of income and health spending, Ghana has weaker health outcomes and fewer inputs (hospital beds and health care workers). Ghana does not appear to get good value for money in terms of health outcomes or high levels of efficiency from its relatively low level of inputs. To more fully understand the system's performance, one must also analyze its financing performance, including the level of financial protection, the fairness/equity of the system, consumer satisfaction, and technical efficiency at the micro level.

Financial parameters. This section provides a global assessment of Ghana's health financing system based on data from the 2009 WHO National Health Accounts (NHA). Although the WHO updates each country's

Figure 2A.23   Total Number of Health Workers per 1,000 People in Ghana and Global Comparator Countries

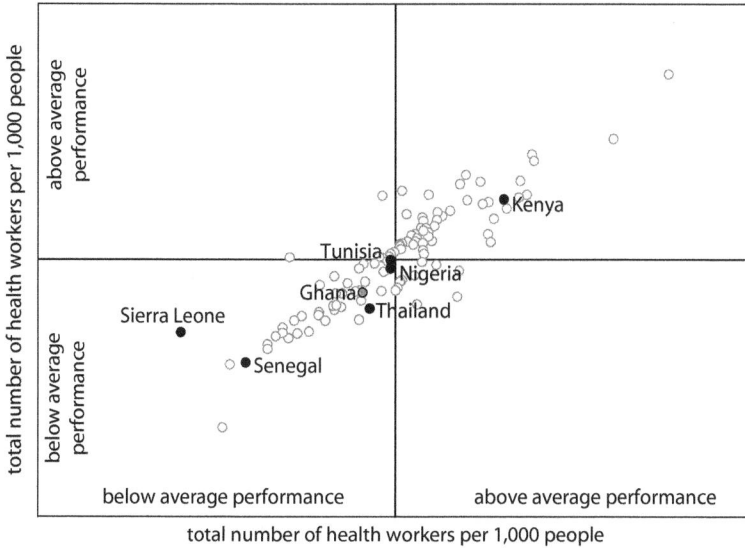

Sources: World Bank 2011b; WHO 2011.
Note: Data are for latest year available 2000–09; health workers include physicians, nurses and midwives, dentists, and pharmacists as well as lower-level cadres.

estimates annually, many of the base parameters used for the estimates come from periodic comprehensive national assessments conducted by countries. Ghana's last comprehensive NHA was performed in 2002. It needs to conduct an updated benchmarking exercise to improve the accuracy of its data and the NHA estimates of the WHO.

Total spending on health. In 2009, total health spending in Ghana was 4.9 percent of GDP, $54 per capita in U.S. dollars, and $125 per capita in international dollars. Ghana's total health spending as a percent of GDP was below the average for countries at its income level (figure 2A.24). Per capita health spending in both exchange rates and international dollars were close to the averages for global comparators (figure 2A.25).

The 2010 GDP revision substantially changed Ghana's relative standing globally. Based on the old GDP figures, Ghana spent almost 8 percent of its GDP on health; the revised GDP estimate reduced this figure to 4.9 percent. Although the per capita figures remained unchanged, per capita spending was above the global averages based on the old GDP figure but close to the global averages based on the new figure. Thus total

Figure 2A.24   Total Health Expenditure as Percent of GDP in Ghana and Global Comparator Countries

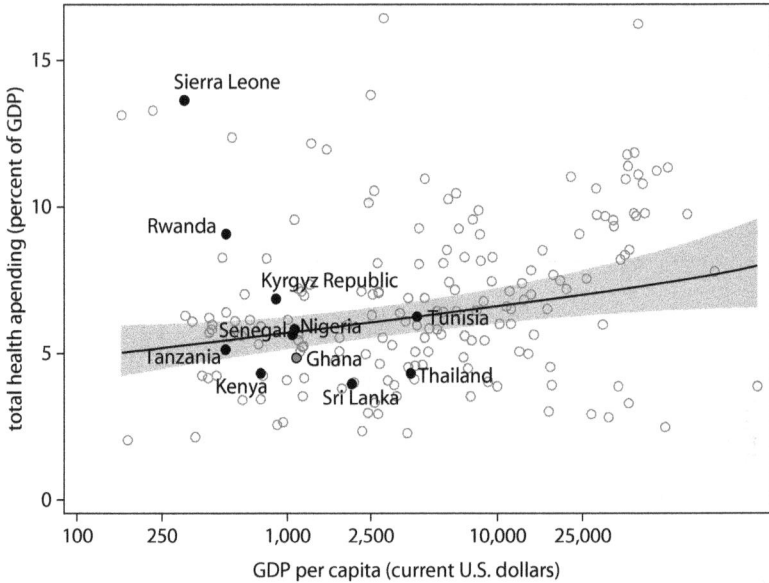

Sources: World Bank 2011b; WHO 2011.
Note: Both axes are log scale.

health spending in Ghana based on these measures appears to be at or slightly below the global averages rather than above average as it was before the revision.

Public spending on health. In 2009, public spending on health in Ghana accounted for 2.6 percent of GDP, 12.6 percent of total government spending, and slightly more than half of total health spending. (Like many other African countries, Ghana spent less than the Abuja target of 15 percent of the government budget on health.) Per capita spending was $29 in U.S. dollars and $66 in international dollars. As a percent of GDP, public spending was about average (figure 2A.26, panel a). As a percent of total government spending, public spending on health was well above average (figure 2A.26, panel b). As a percent of total spending on health, public spending was above average (figure 2A.26, panel c). Per capita public spending was also average (figure 2A.27). As in the case of total spending, these results contrast sharply with the situation before the GDP revision, when Ghana's public spending on health was above the global averages on most of these measures.

Figure 2A.25   Total Per Capita Health Expenditure in Ghana and Global Comparator Countries

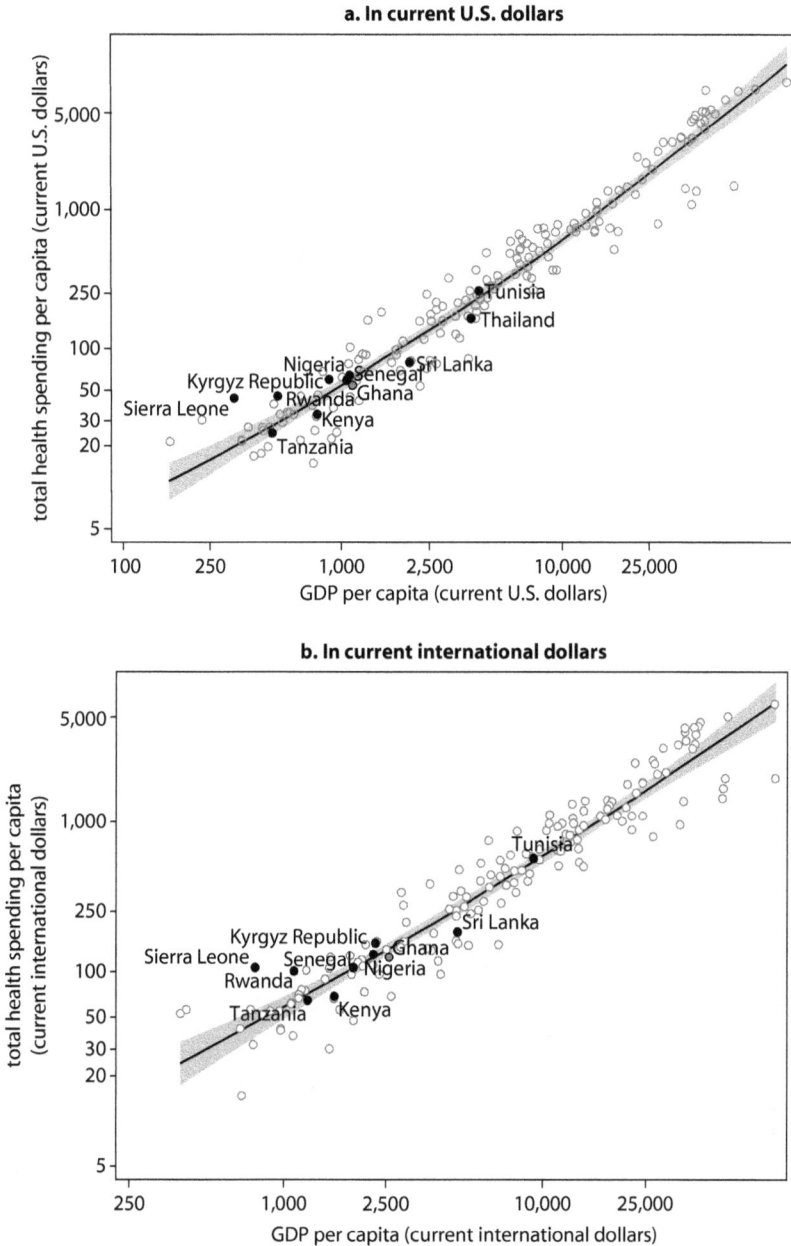

a. In current U.S. dollars

b. In current international dollars

Sources: World Bank 2011b; WHO 2011.
Note: Both axes are log scale.

Figure 2A.26   Public Expenditure on Health in Ghana and Global Comparator Countries

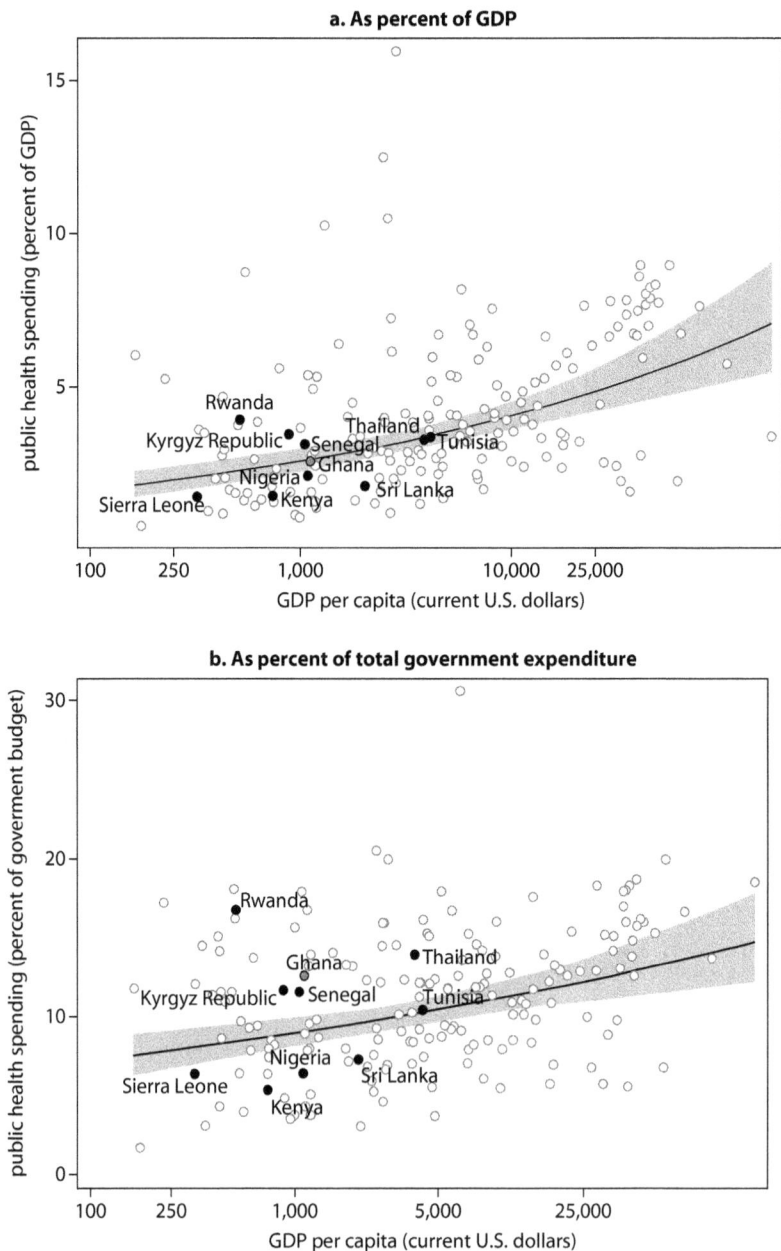

a. As percent of GDP

b. As percent of total government expenditure

(continued next page)

Figure 2A.26   *(continued)*

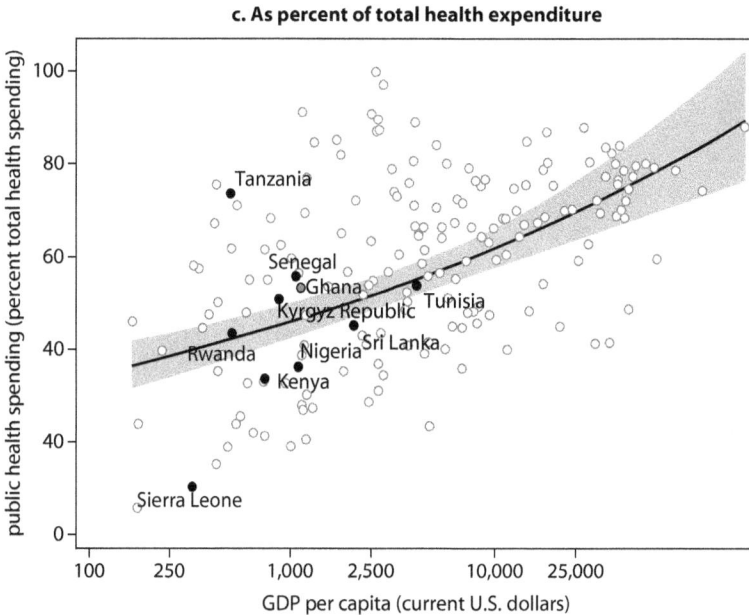

c. As percent of total health expenditure

Sources: World Bank 2011b; WHO 2011.
Note: Both axes are log scale.

Private spending on health. Private spending levels and trends are especially important because they have critical implications for financial protection and the fairness/equity of the system. As countries develop and expand health insurance coverage, private spending as a share of total health spending declines as government health spending increases. Of particular importance is out-of-pocket spending, which directly affects households' financial status.

Private spending in Ghana accounted for 2.3 percent of GDP and slightly less than half of all health spending (figure 2A.28). Per capita private spending was $25 in U.S. dollars and $59 per capita in international dollars, about average for countries at its income level (figure 2A.29).

Overall government spending and revenue effort. Despite Ghana's commitment to poverty reduction and the NHIS, its government spending and revenues were well below global averages (figures 2A.30 and 2A.31). Given its very low revenues, it spends less overall and about

Figure 2A.27   Public Health Expenditure Per Capita in Ghana and Global Comparator Countries

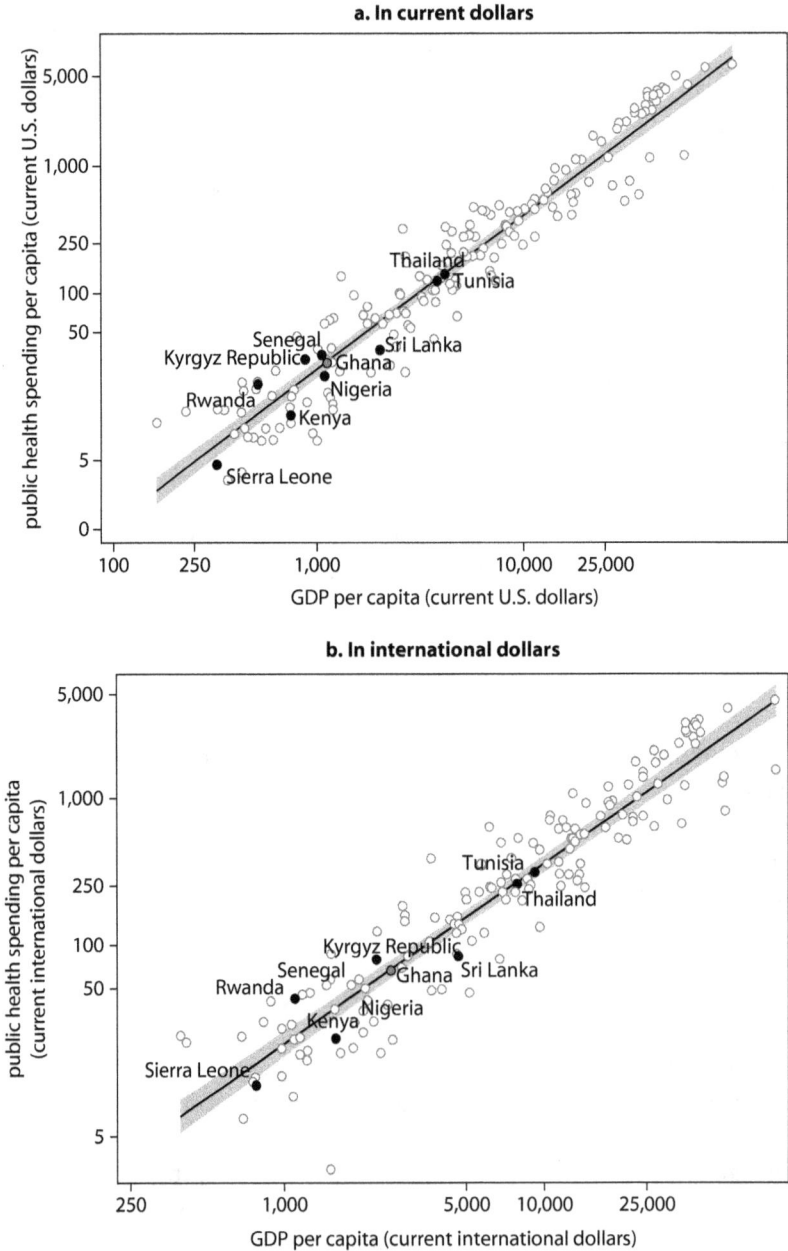

a. In current dollars

b. In international dollars

Sources: World Bank 2011b; WHO 2011.
Note: Both axes are log scale.

Figure 2A.28   Private Health Spending in Ghana and Global Comparator Countries

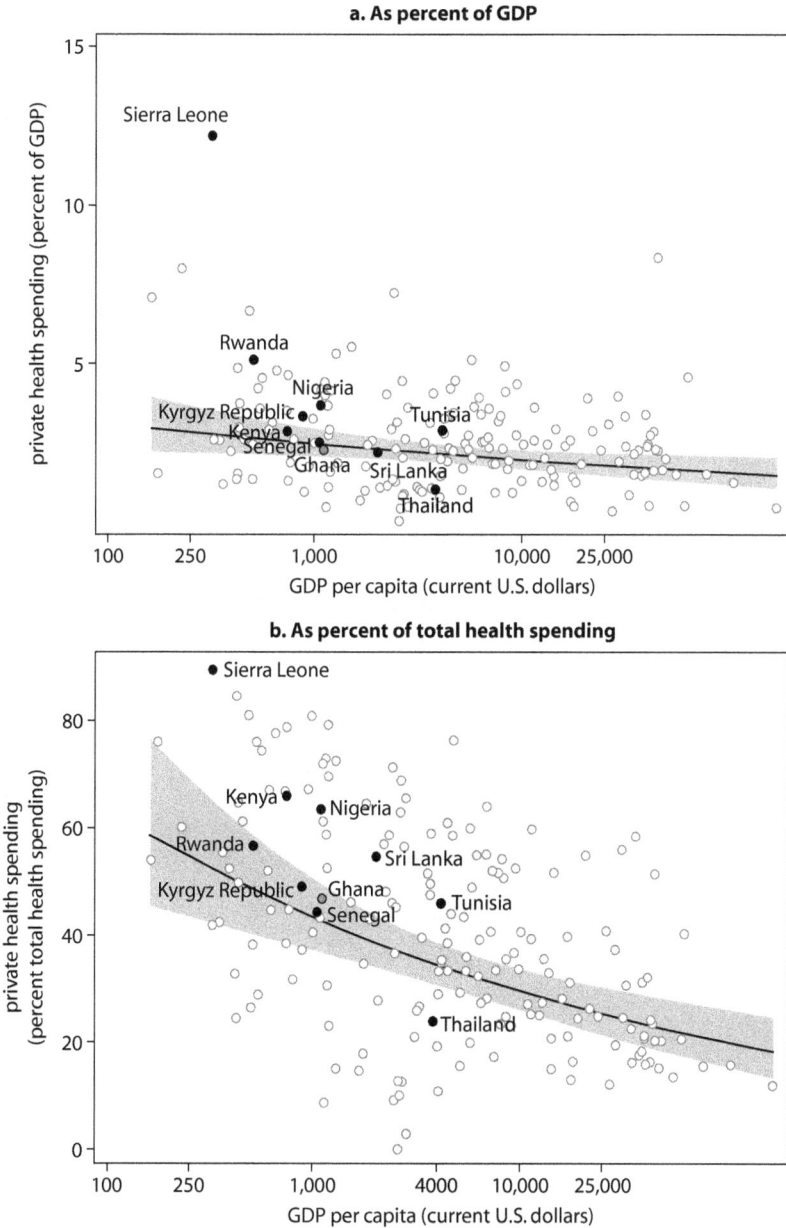

a. As percent of GDP

b. As percent of total health spending

Sources: World Bank 2011b; WHO 2011.
Note: Both axes are log scale.

Figure 2A.29   Private Per Capita Health Expenditure in Ghana and Global Comparator Countries

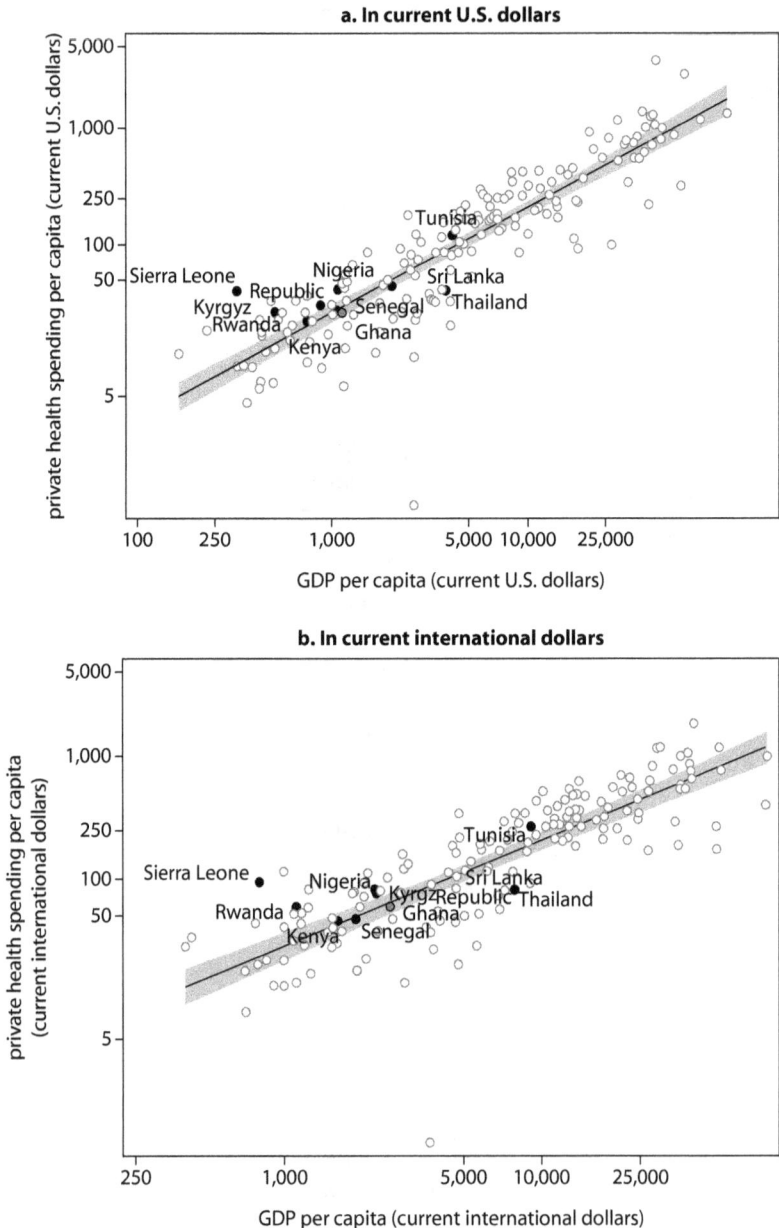

a. In current U.S. dollars

b. In current international dollars

Sources: World Bank 2011b; WHO 2011.
Note: Both axes are log scale.

Figure 2A.30   Total Government Expenditure as Percent of GDP in Ghana and Global Comparator Countries

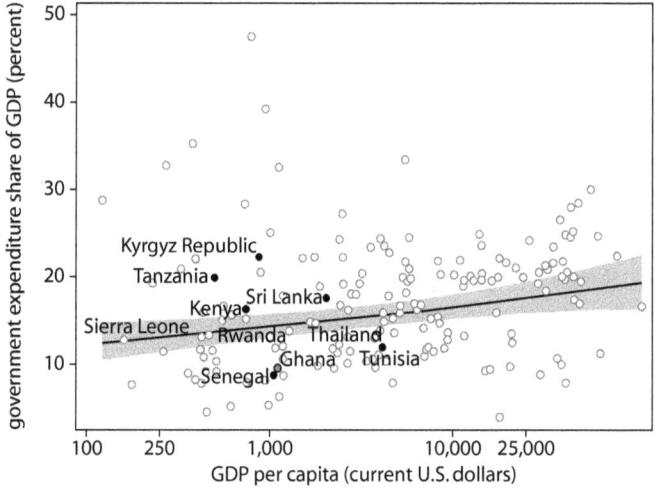

Sources: World Bank 2011b; WHO 2011.
Note: Both axes are log scale. Data are for latest available year 2000–09.

Figure 2A.31   Total Government Revenue as Percent of GDP in Ghana and Global Comparator Countries

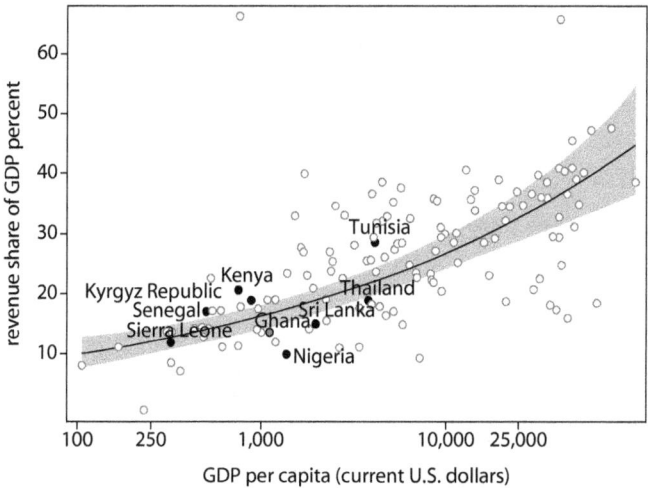

Sources: World Bank 2011b; WHO 2011.
Note: Both axes are log scale. Data are for latest available year 2000–09.

the same on health as other countries with comparable revenue efforts (figure 2A.32). Moreover, as a low-income country, Ghana received significant donor support. It receives average levels of donor support relative to its income comparators, a situation that may not continue now that is has achieved lower-middle-income country status (figure 2A.33).

Equity and financial protection. Out-of-pocket spending is a gross measure of financial protection. In its recent World Health Report (WHO 2010), the WHO argues that when countries reduce out-of-pocket shares to below 15–20 percent of total health spending, their citizens benefit from significant financial protection. Ghana's 37 percent share, although not unusual for a country of its income level, is twice this amount.

Out-of-pocket spending on health accounted for 79 percent of private health spending and 37 percent of total health in Ghana in 2009,

Figure 2A.32 Government Total and Health Spending as Percent of GDP in Ghana and Global Comparator Countries

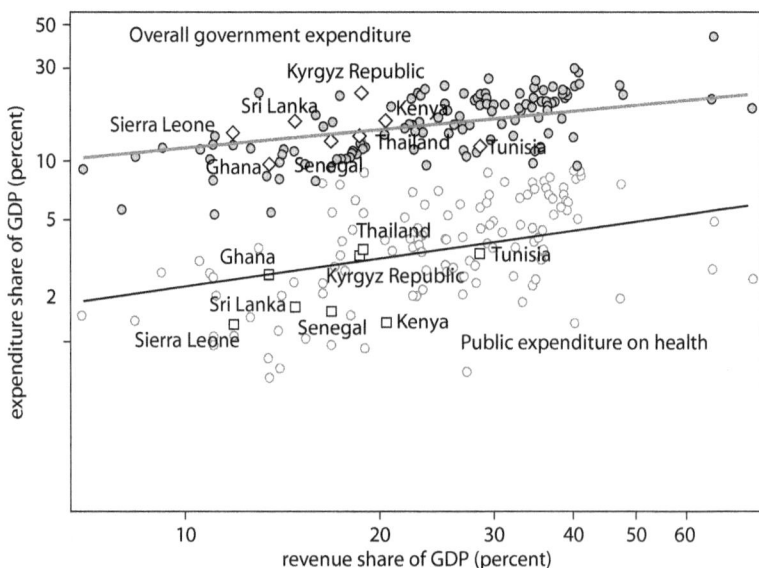

Sources: World Bank 2011b; WHO 2011.
Note: Both axes are log scale. Data are for latests available year 2000–09.

Figure 2A.33   External Assistance as Percent of Total Health Spending in Ghana and Global Comparator Countries

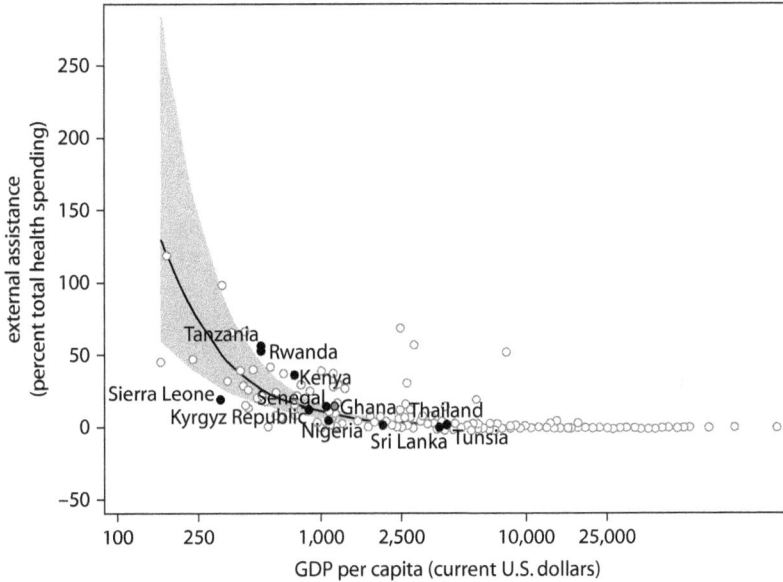

Sources: World Bank 2011b; WHO 2011.
Note: Both axes are log scale.

levels that were at or slightly above the levels of its global comparators (figure 2A.34). Out-of-pocket spending per capita was at the global average (figure 2A.35). Financial protection was thus about or slightly below average. Based on the WHO's 15–20 percent out-of-pocket criterion, however, financial protection in Ghana was insufficient.

Figure 2A.34   Out-of-Pocket Spending on Health in Ghana and Global Comparator Countries

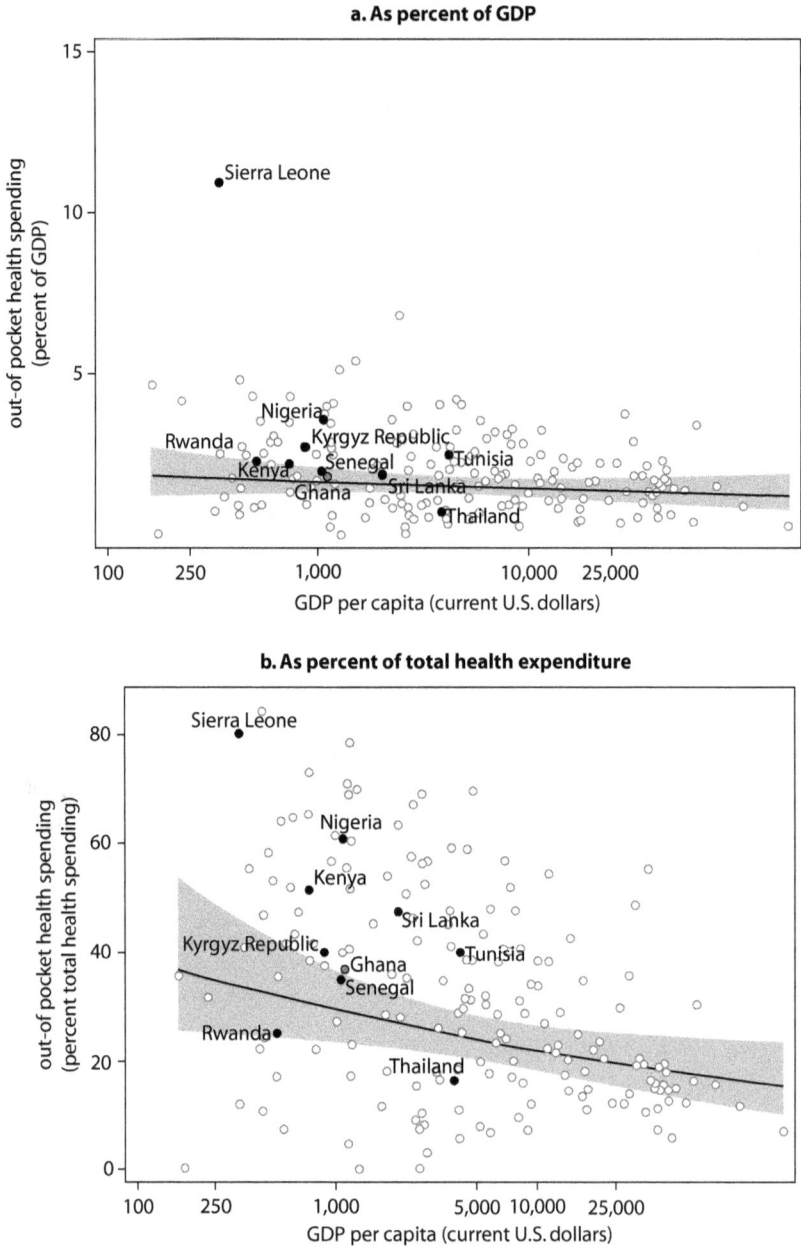

a. As percent of GDP

b. As percent of total health expenditure

Sources: World Bank 2011b; WHO 2011.
Note: Both axes are log scale.

Figure 2A.35   Per Capita Out-of-Pocket Health Expenditure in Ghana and Global Comparator Countries

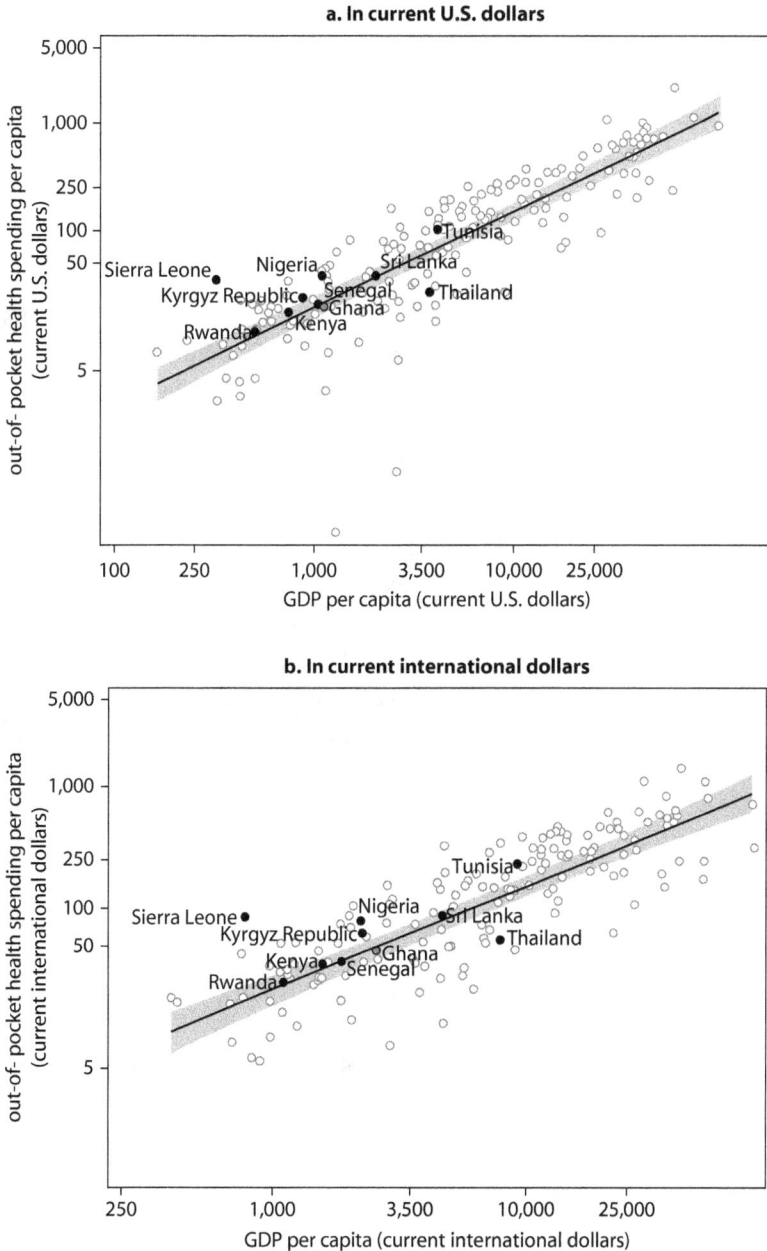

a. In current U.S. dollars

b. In current international dollars

Sources: World Bank 2011b; WHO 2011.
Note: Both axes are log scale.

Notes

1. The lower poverty line captures the amount needed to meet basic nutritional requirements; people falling below this line are in extreme poverty. The upper poverty line includes both essential food and nonfood consumption; people falling above this line are able to purchase essential food and nonfood needs (GSS 2007).

2. SHIELD (Strategies for Health Insurance for Equity in Less Developed Countries) evaluates inequities in health systems in Ghana, South Africa, and Tanzania and examines the extent to which insurance can address them.

3. In preliminary findings from a World Bank report (World Bank 2012) using the older 2005/06 data, which reflect only the beginning of implementation of the NHIS, taxes and social insurance contributions are found to be mildly progressive, voluntary premiums progressive, and out-of-pocket payments slightly regressive. Combining all these effects, they conclude that overall health care financing in Ghana is proportional to income.

4. The study used a purposive sampling of 803 patients in the Komenda-Edina-Eguafo-Abrem district to understand consumer impressions of health service delivery in rural Ghana. Providers included one community clinic, four health centers/posts/clinics, two private maternity homes, one private hospital, and one specialist hospital for skin problems.

5. Options included private providers, public providers, pharmacists, sellers of over-the-counter drugs, traditional/faith healers, and self-treatment.

6. See GHS (2009) for a detailed assessment of Ghana's health system inputs.

7. The results are similar for infant mortality. The results for infant, under-five, and maternal mortality as well as life expectancy are not sensitive to whether U.S. or international dollars are used.

References

Akazili, J., J. Gyapong, and D. McIntyre. 2011. "Who Pays for Health Care in Ghana?" *International Journal for Equity in Health* 10 (26). http://www.equi tyhealthj.com/content/10/1/26.

GHS (Ghana Health Service). 2009. *The Health Sector in Ghana Facts and Figures 2009*. Accra.

GSS (Ghana Statistical Service). 1997. *Core Welfare Indicators Questionnaire*. Accra.

———. 2003. *Core Welfare Indicators Questionnaire*. Accra.

———. 2007. *Patterns and Trends of Poverty in Ghana 1991–2006*. Accra.

———. 2008. *Ghana Living Standards Survey Report of the Fifth Round (GLSS5)*. Accra.

GSS (Ghana Statistical Service), GHS (Ghana Health Service), and ICF Macro. 2009. *Ghana Demographic and Health Survey 2008*. Accra.

GSS (Ghana Statistical Service), NMIMR (Noguchi Memorial Institute for Medical Research), and ORC Macro. 2004. *Ghana Demographic and Health Survey 2003*. Calverton, MD.

Gottret, P., G. Schieber, and H. Waters. 2008. *Good Practices in Health Financing*. World Bank, Washington, DC.

Hendriks, R. 2010. "National Health Insurance Ghana." World Bank, Washington, DC, and Ghana Ministry of Health, Accra.

IMF (International Monetary Fund). 2011a. *Ghana: 2011 Article IV Consultation*. Washington, DC.

———. 2011b. *Staff Report for the 2011 Article IV Consultation*. Africa Department Washington, DC.

Nakamura H., N. Ikeda, A. Stickley, R. Mori, and K. Shibuya. 2011. "Achieving MDG 4 in Sub-Saharan Africa: What Has Contributed to the Accelerated Child Mortality Decline in Ghana?" *PLoS ONE* 6(3).

NDPC (National Development Planning Commission). 2009. *2008 Citizens' Assessment Survey*. NDPC: Accra.

Nketsiah-Amponsah, E. 2009. "Determinants of Consumer Satisfaction of Health Care in Ghana: Does Choice of Health Care Provider Matter?" *Global Journal of Health Science* 1 (2): 50–61.

OECD (Organization for Economic Cooperation and Development). 2010. *Value for Money in Health Spending*. Paris.

Saleh, Karima. Forthcoming (2012). *The Health Sector in Ghana: A Comprehensive Assessment*. Washington, DC: World Bank.

Turkson, P. K. 2009. "Perceived Quality of Healthcare Delivery in a Rural District of Ghana." *Ghana Medical Journal* 43 (2): 65–70.

UNDP (United Nations Development Programme). 2010. *2008 Ghana Millennium Development Goals Report*. New York: UNDP.

Van Doorslaer, E., O. O'Donnell, R. Rannan-Eliya, A. Somanatha, S. Adhikari, C. Garg, D. Harbianto, A. Herrin, M. Huq, and S. Ibragimo. 2007. "Catastrophic Payments for Health Care in Asia." *Health Economics* 16 (11): 1159–84.

WHO (World Health Organization) 2010. *Health Systems Financing: The Path to Universal Coverage*. Geneva: WHO.

———. 2011. *National Health Accounts Data Base*. Geneva. http://apps.who.int/nha/database/PreDataExplorer.aspx?d=1. Accessed November 15, 2011.

World Bank. 2011a. *Republic of Ghana: Joint Review of Public Expenditure and Financial Management.* Africa Region, Washington, DC.

———. 2011b. *World Development Indicators.* Washington, DC.

———. 2012. "Health Equity and Financial Protection Report—Ghana." World Bank, Washington, DC.

CHAPTER 3

Strengths and Weaknesses of Ghana's Health System

This study assesses Ghana's health financing system performance in terms of how well it performs its basic health financing functions (collecting revenue, pooling risk, and purchasing services); improves health outcomes; provides financial protection; and demonstrates consumer responsiveness in an equitable, efficient, and sustainable manner. As health financing interacts with all the other aspects of health systems—as well as other institutions and factors outside the health sector that affect health—assessment of strengths and weaknesses must deal with all aspects of the health system, not only its financing. This chapter does so, based on the performance assessment in chapter 2 and a review of the extensive body of health policy literature on Ghana, including the Country Status Report (Saleh forthcoming [2012]) and the background papers prepared for it. The body of the chapter summarizes the main findings; annex 3A presents the full results.

Strengths and weaknesses are classified into three broad categories: governance, management, and organization; delivery system, pharmaceuticals, and public health; and financing. There is no single "right" taxonomy, and as in all health systems classifications, most of the elements interact both within and across the three broad categories.

The analysis in this chapter is based on an extensive review of the rich literature on Ghana, which includes the following sources:

- the government's Health Sector Medium Term Development Plan
- major donor reports (for example, IHP+ 2010; Smith and Fairbank 2008)
- the World Bank's 2011 Public Expenditure Review, the Ghana Country Status Report (CSR) (Saleh forthcoming [2012]), and the numerous background papers for the CSR (Couttolenc 2012; Dubbeldam and others 2011; Sealy, Makinen, and Bitran 2011; Seiter 2011; Appiah and others forthcoming).
- the Ghana case study for the World Bank Institute's 2010 Health Reform Flagship Course (Nyonator 2010a, b, and c)
- the 2010 and 2011 annual reports of the National Health Insurance Authority (NHIA)
- a report on the National Health Insurance Scheme (NHIS) by the World Bank and the Ministry of Health (World Bank and Ghana Ministry of Health 2009)
- the background paper on Ghana for the 2010 *World Health Report* of the World Health Organization (WHO) (Durairaj, D'Almeida, and Kirigia 2010)
- OXFAM's critique of the coverage of Ghana's health insurance scheme (Apoya and Marriott 2011)
- an actuarial technical assistance report on Ghana's health insurance scheme (Hendriks 2010)
- the recent report on Ghana's health insurance system by the Rockefeller Foundation (Seddoh, Adjei, and Nazzar 2011)
- the recent report by Akazili, Gyapong, and McIntyre (2011) on the health financing arrangements of Ghana and the NHIS.

Governance, Management, and Organization

Ghana has a well-developed, highly decentralized, and evolving health system. The government is committed to health and has developed an integrated three-level (national, regional, and district) health system that incorporates a community-level health delivery system. Its governance, management, and organization reflect this structure.

The system has significant strengths:

- The government has put in place the administrative and legal requirements for its decentralized governance structure.

- The public financial management system is adequate, clear, and meets most international requirements.
- Successive common management arrangements provide an effective framework for relating to partners.
- The NHIS legislation (Act 650) strategically sets out an elaborate governance and administrative framework for the provision of health insurance.
- The level of consumer satisfaction is high.

The system still faces some major challenges, however, which hinder effective management and operation:

- There are potential inconsistencies between the government's overall decentralization model of devolution and the Ghana Health Service's model of deconcentration.
- Local authorities have little control over budgets and expenditures, because most of their resources are executed centrally or earmarked from the center to specific programs or initiatives.
- Health workforce ratios are weak; health infrastructure, equipment, and transport deficits are large; the Health Management Information System (HMIS) has major deficiencies; drug procurement and the performance of the central medical stores with respect to financing, quality assurance, and logistics management are weak.
- Poor coordination among the various regulatory agencies results in high drug prices and substandard drugs.

These problems represent serious challenges to the equitable and efficient functioning of the health financing system overall as well as the coverage, payment, quality assurance, and provider certification operations of the NHIS. The government is well aware of these challenges and is attempting to deal with them through various planning processes.

Delivery System, Pharmaceuticals, and Public Health

Improving health outcomes, financial protection, and consumer responsiveness in an equitable, efficient, and sustainable manner requires a well-functioning delivery system of human and physical infrastructure; reasonably priced, available, and effective pharmaceuticals (which represented 40–50 percent of all NHIS spending in 2008 [Seiter 2011]); and well-functioning public health programs that target the major disease burdens (for example, malaria, noncommunicable diseases) and are tightly coordinated with the NHIS basic benefits package. Ghana has come a long way in terms of developing a modern health care delivery system, improving the availability of effective drugs, and operating effective public health programs.

The strengths of these systems include the following:

- There have been large increases in human resources for health and production of nurses; Ghana produces more doctors than many countries in the region.
- Since the 2006 salary increase, exits from the labor market have been largely a result of retirement, not outmigration.
- Informal payments are reportedly uncommon.
- The Ministry of Health and the Ghana Health Service have developed a comprehensive approach to set priorities for investments, considering recurrent costs, human resource constraints, maintenance implications, and other factors.
- Outpatient department utilization has increased significantly.
- Overall hospital use trends for most categories are positive, with occupancy rates increasing from 45 percent to 60 percent and average lengths of stay decreasing from 4.5 to 3.8 days between 2005 and 2009.
- A vibrant private sector is a major care supplier of all forms of nonhospital care and a significant supplier of hospital care.
- Ghana has a reasonable essential drugs list and good availability of drugs.
- Full immunization coverage has increased, HIV/AIDS prevalence is low, and Ghana is likely to meet the Millennium Development Goal (MDG) target for child nutrition.

Like all countries, Ghana also faces serious challenges in the equity, efficiency, and overall performance of its service delivery system, pharmaceutical system, and public health programs. These challenges include the following:

- Current health care provider densities are far below the levels recommended by the World Health Organization (WHO).
- There are too few health workers, and their regional distribution favors urban areas, especially for high-level cadres. Too few health workers are assigned to areas with high levels of poverty.
- There are few incentives to ensure good performance by health workers.

- Hospital occupancy rates are just 60 percent, and there is considerable interregional variation in occupancy, beds, average lengths of stay, and turnover.
- Expansion of health infrastructure is limited by inadequate financial resources; delays in the release of budgetary allocations, resulting in cost overruns; unplanned initiation of projects outside the capital investment plan; weak planned preventive maintenance; and issues with the acquisition, distribution, installation, and use of equipment.
- There is a need to strengthen district health and subdistrict health systems, with a focus on primary care.
- Ghana is unlikely to meet the MDG targets for child and maternal mortality; anemia is a major problem among women and children; the use of contraceptives is low and stagnant, with high levels of unmet need; and the prevalence of tuberculosis is high and stagnant, with high levels of unmet needs.

Many of these challenges are common in lower-income countries; they are exacerbated in a geographically diverse country like Ghana.

To achieve its health reform goals, Ghana must deal with the inefficiencies and inequities in its service delivery system and do a much better job of providing primary care. Better performance of its health programs is essential; these programs need to be realigned to deal with both the significant communicable disease burden and the increasing burden of noncommunicable diseases and injuries. Doing so will require better coordination of these programs with the NHIS basic benefits package.

Pharmaceuticals are both an important determinant of health outcomes and impoverishment and a major cost driver in the system. Ensuring equity, efficiency and effectiveness in the availability and use of pharmaceuticals is critical to improving health outcomes and controlling costs.

Health Financing

Health financing interacts with all aspects of health systems. A well-designed and functioning health financing system is therefore critical.

Ghana's health financing system has several notable strengths:

- Ghana is one of very few emerging market countries to take serious steps toward demand-side financing of health, pass legislation for universal health insurance coverage, begin implementing it by covering vulnerable groups while significantly expanding enrollment, and ear-marking substantial resources to support the system.

- The revenue base for Ghana's overall health financing system is largely progressive, and the NHIS relies on a diversified set of largely progressive funding sources, resulting in significant and stable sources of revenues.
- Ghana's approach is pragmatically built on its existing system of com-munity-based health insurance plans, which transitioned into district mutual health insurance schemes (DMHISs). It is evolving toward a uniform national system.
- According to the NHIS, membership has steadily increased to 8.16 million active members in 2010, some 34 percent of the popu-lation. Between 2005 and 2008, outpatient visits increased by a fac-tor of 23, inpatient service by factor of 29, and expenditures by a factor of 40 (Hendriks 2010).

Ghana is in its early stages of implementing the NHIS. Given the 10–15 years it has taken most other emerging market counties to fully scale up, it is not surprising that NHIS authorities face many critical challenges and the need to make both structural and operational midcourse corrections. The main challenges they need to address include the following:

- With current expenditure and expansion plans, the NHIS is not finan-cially viable. It is projected to be insolvent by as early as 2013.
- Premiums, taxes, and reinsurance payments for the NHIS and to DMHISs are not actuarially determined, and premiums for informal sector workers are low relative to their costs.
- The original health insurance law does not require a necessary reserve fund.
- The basic benefits package is heavily biased toward curative care, coor-dination with Ministry of Health vertical programs is poor, and cover-age of 95 percent of the burden of disease with no cost sharing may not be affordable.
- Lack of effective gatekeeper and referral systems and misaligned pro-vider payment incentives preclude the NHIS from being an effective "active" purchaser.
- Large numbers (perhaps on the order of 30 percent) of the 65 percent of NHIS members, who are exempt from paying premiums, could afford to contribute. Meanwhile, the stringent definition of indigent excludes some poor and near poor.

- Lack of a modern HMIS results in poor claims management and quality assurance, high administrative costs, and incomplete information on enrollees and providers.

Although the focus of this study is on the NHIS, Ghanaian policy makers also need to focus holistically on the financing of the entire health system, including the Ministry of Health, the Ghana Health Service, and private financing. The NHIS is a critical focal point, because as coverage expands, it will become the largest payer for health care services. Its role raises important policy decisions. Will the public delivery system evolve into autonomous entities? Will public sector health workers continue to be salaried government employees? What will the government's future role be in the direct provision of care? What will be the roles and responsibilities of the national versus local governments as regulators as opposed to providers—will the national government steer the ship or be the ship?

As discussed in the government's various planning documents and the Country Status Report (Saleh forthcoming [2012]), Ghana is grappling with these interrelated management, delivery system, and financing issues. Chapter 4 provides an overview of the future fiscal context that overlays these policy choices. Chapter 5 discusses specific health financing reform options based on this assessment of strengths and weaknesses.

Annex 3A. Detailed Analysis of the Strengths and Weaknesses of Ghana's Health System

This annex assesses the strengths and weaknesses of Ghana's health system in terms of three broad categories of health systems features: governance, management, and organization; delivery system, pharmaceuticals, and public health; and, health financing. As noted, there is no "right" taxonomy to classify health systems; the numerous health systems elements can be classified under more than one heading, and most elements interact across categories. This annex describes the key elements, their interactions, and their ultimate impacts on the performance of the health system. Recognizing that health systems are extremely complex and dynamic organisms, the purpose here is to get a snapshot of the key performance parameters, irrespective of how one categorizes them.

A few important caveats are in order. First, the assessment is based on the latest available government and development partner documents, recent studies, and data. Many aspects of performance (for example, unit cost information on efficiency and recent household data on consumption and spending), data are lacking. The most recent studies available are often based on dated information. Second, the NHIS recently made some major changes (offering free maternal care and waiving waiting periods for certain groups, for example), which the studies cited in this annex do not reflect. Finally, as with any assessment of strengths and weaknesses, one can view a glass as half full or half empty. Certain strengths also have elements of weaknesses. For example, significant progress has been made in reforming financial management, but it still falls short of full compliance with agreed upon standards.

Governance, Management, and Organization
Strengths

- The government has spent 30 years putting in place the administrative and legal requirements for its decentralized governance structure.

- The public financial management system is adequate and clear, it meets most international requirements, and the government is committed to reforms to further improve its effectiveness (World Bank 2011).

- The government is committed to health and has developed an integrated three-level health system (national, regional, and district). The subdistrict level includes a community health delivery system focused on access, quality, and coverage of health information; preventive care; clinical care; and emergency services.

- In addition to legal frameworks, successive common management arrangements (built on sectorwide approaches, the Paris Declaration of Aid Effectiveness, and so forth) provide a framework within which public sector actors interact with various partners in the health sector to ensure the principles of one country plan; budget and reporting mechanism; support for country-led approaches to health development; the strengthening of financing and systems; and a common monitoring and evaluation framework for all stakeholders.

- Act 650 sets out an elaborate governance and administrative set-up for the NHIS and establishes schemes that are protected within the existing Ministry of Health and local government structures, empowering districts, within central government guidelines, to govern the delivery of health services by contracting with providers.[1]

Weaknesses

- Across sectors, most government revenue in Ghana goes to labor (57 percent in 2008), leaving few resources for goods, services, and investment. The health sector accounted for 13 percent of public employment in 2008; salaries for public sector health workers accounted for 55 percent of recurrent Ministry of Health spending.

- A regular and comprehensive review of public expenditure, from an effectiveness, efficiency and sustainability perspective, is lacking (domestically financed public investment projects are not based on careful cost-benefit analysis and the computation of financial and social economic returns). Transparency, executive accountability, and oversight of public financial management are weak.

- An effective decentralized health sector faces a number of serious challenges. The main problem is that the government's overall model of decentralization is devolution (the shifting of responsibility/authority from the central office of the Ministry of Health to separate public administrative structures, such as local governments), whereas the basic approach of the Ghana Health Service is deconcentration (the shifting of power from the central office to peripheral offices of the same administration). Other issues include the low levels of control local authorities have over budget and expenditure and the fact that most of the resources allocated to local facilities and services are actually executed centrally on behalf of local offices or earmarked from the center to specific programs or initiatives.

- Making decentralization work requires the following:
  - systematic assessment of district health administrations and district assemblies
  - a single legal framework for health system decentralization
  - stronger linkages between top-down and bottom-up health planning
  - stronger stewardship/leadership roles of the Ministry of Health and local governments as well as greater local government capacity
  - monitoring and evaluation of the decentralization process and the stewardship role of the Ministry of Health

- a financing framework for local governments using the district financing fund to consolidate flows and practical guidelines for "composite budgets"
- modified procurement processes to standardize processes at different government levels
- intersectoral and multisectoral action to achieve health gains.
- Strategies regarding all aspects of the development and implementation of supply-side management policies (policy development; regulation and inspection; supply management; rational use of medicines) are lacking:
  - There is no well-articulated quality assurance system in place for the management of procurement and supplies to ensure health commodity security at all levels and facilities.
  - The multiplicity of procurement and supply chains (central medical stores, the NHIA, Ghana Health Service budget management centers, faith-based organizations) should be replaced by a single central procurement agency.
  - There is no monitoring or supervision of faith-based health organizations.
  - There is no national institutional framework for regulating laboratories or imaging centers.
  - Elements for the implementation of the essential medicines policy are lacking.
- Government oversight of the public and private sector delivery systems is weak, and involvement of the for-profit private sector is too limited.
- Although significant progress has been made in health services planning, standardization of designs for specific facilities, equipment maintenance, and other aspects of the health system, problems persist:
  - Capital planning is complex. It takes place in an environment in which priority setting is often heavily influenced by nontechnical arguments issues, such as political intervention. Funding comes from a large number of sources, often with conditionalities.
  - Management is weak. For example, there is no systematic record-keeping on the overall level of capital investments.
  - Identification of new projects is incomplete as a result of the many different avenues for approval and funding.
  - The "split" between the Ministry of Health and the Ghana Health Services leads to a lack of clarity on the division of labor with regard to several planning and management functions.
  - Coordination of capital planning with other stakeholders in the health sector is suboptimal. In certain districts, for example, public

district hospitals are being projected even though the Christian Health Association of Ghana is already operating functional district hospitals.

- A national information and communication technology strategy has not been developed for the health sector, and the HMIS is weak at all levels (World Bank 2007).
- Managerial autonomy and capacity is lacking at the facility level, and the standardization of human resource management policies is weak.
- Although targeting has improved recently, particularly in programs like Livelihood Empowerment Against Poverty (LEAP), substantial room remains for improvement in many other programs through the use of a common targeting mechanism (for example, for LEAP, the NHIS, and the school uniforms programs).
- Many NHIA organizational and managerial difficulties stem from the original institutional framework of the NHIS legislation (Nyonator 2010a,b, and c; Seddoh, Adjei, and Nazzar 2011):
  - The legal and institutional framework for running independent, autonomous, and decentralized DMHISs has yielded a system without appropriate layers of administrative and financial oversight, clear lines of supervision, or due process.
  - Although the DMHISs depend on the NHIA for most of their funding, including bailouts, they assert their legal and operational independence over issues of accountability to the authority for funding received and general oversight. As a result, some DMHISs are encountering serious governance, institutional, operational, administrative, and financial problems, and in some areas they are unable to meet their fundamental object of providing access to health care services for their clients.

Like many countries with highly decentralized governance and administrative structures (for example, Indonesia, the Philippines), Ghana faces many difficult legal, fiscal, and administrative issues in ensuring effective functioning of a very complex sector. Indeed, there are contradictions in the basic models of decentralization between the government's basic devolution approach and the Ghana Health Service's deconcentration modus operandi. For its part, the NHIS is in the process of national standardization and recentralization of its administrative and operational functions. These varied approaches may make sense in their individual contexts (for example, economies of scale and standardization in NHIS enrollment, revenue collection, claims processing, and provider payment).

However, ensuring that the legal, regulatory, administrative, and fiscal structures support effective implementation of these various approaches is a major challenge. Without effective information for decision making, operational frameworks (including frameworks for eliminating corruption), and appropriate incentives, health financing reform efforts are doomed to failure.

Delivery System, Pharmaceuticals, and Public Health

The WHO framework for characterizing health systems contains six principal elements: service delivery; health workforce; information; medical products, vaccines, and technologies; health financing; and leadership/governance. Leadership/governance was discussed in the previous section; health financing is discussed in the next section. The focus here is on the other health systems elements as well as their critical sub-elements (for example, physical infrastructure, public health, medicines).

Strengths
Overall performance

- Ghana has a well-developed, integrated, multilevel health system, composed of community-based health planning and services; health centers; district, regional, and teaching hospitals; private health providers; and nongovernmental health-related organizations.
- The level of consumer satisfaction is high.
- Access to care has increased, with 64 percent of the ill obtaining care in 2005, up from 44 percent in 1999.
- Ghana has a reasonable essential drugs list and good availability of drugs.
- All of the government's proposed interventions for disease prevention and control are based on evidence and Ghana's robust experience with public health programs.

Human resources for health

- The number of health workers has increased, as has the production of nurses.
- The production of doctors is higher than in many countries in the region.
- Since the 2006 salary increase, exits from the labor market have been largely a result of retirement, not outmigration. As a result of that

change, wages in the sector are higher than wages in other sectors in Ghana. They are also higher than wages of health workers elsewhere in Africa.

- Absenteeism appears to be limited.
- Informal payments are not reported to be common.[2]

Infrastructure

- The Ministry of Health and the Ghana Health Service have developed comprehensive approaches to set priorities for investments, considering "systems" variables, such as recurrent cost implications, human resource constraints, and maintenance implications.
- Outpatient department utilization has increased significantly since 2001. For the period between 2004 and 2009, overall hospital use trends for most categories were positive. The bed occupancy rate rose from 45 percent to 60 percent, and the average length of stay fell from 4.5 to 3.8 days.
- A vibrant private sector is a major supplier of all forms of nonhospital care and a significant supplier of hospital care in several districts, largely in urban areas. It produces more than half of all services used in virtually every category.

Public health

- Full immunization coverage has increased, the prevalence of HIV/AIDS is low, and Ghana is likely to meet the child nutrition MDG target.

Weaknesses
Overall performance

- Among countries with similar levels of income and health spending, Ghana performs worse than average with respect to under-five (and infant) and maternal mortality, and it will fall short of achieving its MDG targets in these areas.
- Over the past several decades, Ghana's improvements in health outcomes have been much less impressive than several neighboring countries', despite starting from better levels.
- Ghana has fewer physicians and health workers per capita than other countries with comparable levels of income and health spending, and it has a serious shortage of specialists.

- In 2009, Ghana had fewer hospital beds per capita than other countries with comparable levels of income and health spending. Its bed occupancy rate was only 60 percent, and geographic disparities were wide, indicating suboptimal allocation and use of hospital beds.
- Over the past several decades, increases in the number of hospital beds and physicians per capita have been smaller than in many neighboring countries. Over the past decade, hospital bed growth has not kept pace with population growth.
- Ghana's integrated health system faces challenges at every level in terms of workforce ratios; infrastructure, equipment, and transport deficits; the collection, analysis, and use of health data; drug procurement and the disappointing performance of the central medical stores; financing; quality assurance; and logistics management.
- Significant changes in the legal framework and regulatory system concerning the roles and responsibilities of the seven health-related regulatory agencies (overseeing public, private, and civil society organizations) are needed in order to ensure better coordination and regulation of services at all levels. Ministry of Health regulatory agencies need sufficient resources to conduct ongoing supervision and monitoring of the private sector.
- Although the government clearly indicates that health gains are to be achieved through primary health care and district health systems, the "systems approach" has not yet translated into a clear approach to strengthening health systems covering all aspects of health system improvement, including issues related to fragmentation ("silofication").
- Access to sanitation is lacking (10 percent versus 34 percent in Sub-Saharan Africa).

Human resources for health. Major changes in human resource policies and implementation are needed to meet the equity challenges posed by the unequal urban-rural distribution of staff (especially high-level cadres), the inadequate total numbers of staff, the inadequate number of health workers in regions with high poverty levels, and the inequitable provision of prenatal care. These challenges require the development of appropriate staffing norms and the effective redeployment of staff, commitment, productivity, and attitude; the decentralization of some aspects of human resource management; and better policies to address housing and infrastructural needs.

- Current health care provider densities are far below WHO recommended levels.

- There are few incentives to ensure the performance of health sector workers.
- Education and training need improvement. The performance of the medical education system is inconsistent; it is particularly weak in rural areas and in the training of rural-inclined students. Policies on producing community health nurses are weak, and there are concerns about overproduction and training expenses. Midwifery training needs expansion. There is little private sector investment in training and production.
- Productivity varies by type of facility and the level of staffing, with high staffing levels associated with lower outputs per worker. Recent increases in the number of health workers and pay have not adequately translated into increased outputs and benefits.
- Leadership and management could be improved by eliminating promotions based on seniority, sanctioning workers for poor performance, and increasing manager empowerment.
- Private sector providers lack access to credit and have poor management skills.
- Health profession and provider associations contribute little to monitoring and ensuring quality of care or developing the business and financial skills of their members.

Infrastructure

- The distribution of existing and new health facilities has been suboptimal. As a result, there is overdevelopment in some locations and underinvestment in others. In addition, publicly provided health services have expanded beyond the limits of available operating funds and professional staffing, resulting in many newly developed facilities being operated with substandard levels of staffing and equipment.
- Hospital occupancy rates are low (60 percent), and there is considerable interregional variation in occupancy, beds, average length of stay, and bed turnover, indicating suboptimal use of the hospital bed stock and the need for much better planning.
- The Ministry of Health/Project Monitoring Unit is underresourced to deal with the rapid increase in the volume of infrastructure work and the completion of legacy projects.
- Financial analysis of capital investments indicates consistent underperformance of reported capital expenditure against budget in recent years.

- District and subdistrict health systems need to be strengthened, with a focus on primary care, particularly at the subdistrict level, where comprehensive primary care services can and should be provided.
- Health infrastructure expansion is limited by the following factors:
  - inadequate financial resources
  - delays in the release of budgetary allocations, resulting in cost overruns
  - unplanned initiation of projects outside the capital investment plan
  - weak planned preventive maintenance
  - problems with the acquisition, distribution, installation, use, and maintenance of equipment. In district hospitals, most equipment is nonfunctional, antiquated, or inadequate; 50–65 percent of all vehicles are over age and need replacement.
- There is a need to strengthen district health and subdistrict health systems, with a focus on primary care, particularly at the subdistrict level, where comprehensive primary care services can and should be provided.
- Although the concept of equipment management is well established in the health sector, implementation of this concept varies:
  - Coverage of equipment support by Ministry of Health appears not to reach the specialized facilities after initial inputs.
  - The location of equipment managers is problematic in some areas and for certain types of facilities.
  - Specialist outreach technical services operated by the clinical engineering department of the Ghana Health Service and the biomedical engineering unit of the Ministry of Health are not very effective.
- Incomplete accreditation of private providers by the NHIS may limit access to private providers.

Public health

- Ghana is unlikely to meet the child and maternal mortality ratio MDG targets; anemia is a major problem among women and children; the contraceptive prevalence rate is low and stagnant, with high levels of unmet need; and the prevalence of tuberculosis is high and stagnant, with large unmet needs.

Other factors

- Poor coordination by regulatory agencies results in high prices for medicines and substandard drugs.

- Demand-side factors appear to be most problematic at the community level and for population-based health services.
- Clinical care coverage is inadequate. Demand- and supply-side factors include the following:
  - Many people lack physical access to primary health care.
  - Staff lack adequate capacity.
  - Maternal and neonatal mortality and nutrition remain big problems. Improving outcomes requires increasing access to an appropriate number of well-performing health workers and better synergy among key institutions (the Ministry of Health, the Ghana Health System, and the NHIS) (El Idrissi 2007).
  - Referral systems are weak.
  - Uptake of assisted deliveries is low.
  - Malaria control is constrained by supply-side constraints: only 49 percent of districts have the long-lasting insecticide treaded nets they need.

Developing, effectively operating, and sustainably financing a health system to achieve basic health system goals is extremely challenging for all countries. It is particularly challenging for low and lower-middle-income countries, which often lack the financing, essential inputs, and technical expertise to implement "good practice" state-of-the-art policies.

Ghana has a well-developed, functional health system throughout the country. It faces many of the same generic problems of underresourcing and maldistribution of resources that most low- and lower-middle-income countries face. For its income and health spending levels, it has fewer inputs than comparators. More troubling is the fact that its health outcomes are generally worse than comparators'. It faces additional challenges as a result of its highly decentralized nature.

The system also has significant strengths. It is vertically integrated; human resources for health production are adequate; absenteeism, outmigration, and informal payments are limited; and consumer (although not workforce) satisfaction and wage levels are high. Utilization has been increasing as the number of health care workers has risen and physical infrastructure improved, although the value for money spent is far from clear. Lack of data for decision making is problematic at all levels of the system.

As NHIS coverage expands to the rest of the population, it is essential for the government to improve the efficiency and effectiveness of the system, deal with maldistribution problems, and expand capacity, including through more effective regulation and better inclusion of the private sector. Capacity expansions will be costly and require additional fiscal space, whether they are financed by the government, the private sector, or the NHIS. Ghana's relatively poor health outcomes, which reflect numerous factors, would suggest the need to reexamine basic public programs and, as discussed below, better coordinate them with the NHIS basic benefits package.

Health Financing

The NHIS has been lauded as an innovative and "good practice" approach to financing health insurance in lower-income settings (see, for example, WHO 2010) and criticized as an inequitable and ineffective failure (see, for example, Apoya and Marriott 2011). Its detailed operational and financial aspects have been assessed, although the assessments have been encumbered by lack of micro-level coverage, claims, and cost information. The analysis that follows focuses on the basic structural design, operational processes, and fiscal features of the NHIS; the performance of its health financing functions in terms of basic health systems objectives; and its long-term financial sustainability, particularly in light of the new macroeconomic realities.

Strengths

- Ghana is one of a very small group of emerging market countries to take serious steps toward demand-side financing for health, pass legislation for universal health insurance coverage, begin implementation by covering vulnerable groups, significantly expand enrollment, and earmark substantial resources to support the system.

- The NHIS relies on a diversified set of funding sources, which has been an important factor in the stability and sustainability of health financing in a number of countries (Kutzin, Jakab, and Cashin 2010).

- The government's commitment to health is evident. Ghana earmarks 2.5 percentage points of the value added tax (VAT) and 2.5 percentage points of the 18.5 percentage point Social Security and National Insurance Trust (SSNIT) tax to the NHIS (these sources accounted for 77 percent of NHIS revenues in 2009). Investments in health infrastructure are also made through concessional loans outside the sector allocation. The 2010 Ghana national budget allows additional employment of staff only for education and health.

- Ghana's approach is pragmatically built on its existing system of community-based health insurance plans, which have evolved into the existing system of DMHISs (some 145 schemes). It is transitioning toward a uniform national system.

- According to the NHIS, membership has steadily increased to 8.16 million active members in 2010.

- Between 2005 and 2008, outpatient visits increased by a factor of 23, inpatient service increased by a factor of 29, and expenditures by increased by a factor of 40.

- The NHIS is funded largely through general government revenues. It uses 2.5 percentage points of the VAT to finance exempt and subsidized groups and deficits of the DMHISs (61 percent of revenues in 2009) and 2.5 percentage points of the 18.5 percentage point SSNIT to finance coverage of public and formal sector workers (15.6 percent). Other sources of revenue included investment income (17 percent), premiums of informal sector workers (3.8 percent), sector budget support (2.3 percent), and other income (0.2 percent).

- Difficult to identify and enroll informal sector employees, who account for 70–90 percent of the workforce and 29 percent of NHIS members, are encouraged to enroll through highly subsidized income-related premiums.

- A 2011 study of the revenue incidence of Ghana's health financing system and the NHIS finds that "Ghana's health care system is generally progressive. The progressivity of financing is driven largely by the overall progressivity of taxes, which account for close to 50 percent of health care funding. The national health insurance (NHI) levy (part of VAT) is mildly progressive and formal sector NHI payroll deductions are also progressive. However, informal sector NHI contributions were found to be regressive. Out-of-pocket payments, which account for 45 percent of funding, are a regressive form of payment to households" (Akazili, Gyapong, and McIntyre 2011).

- As shown in chapter 2, recent studies of the benefit incidence suggest that the program benefits the lower income quintiles but that its targeting could be improved.

- A comprehensive basic benefits package covers some 95 percent of Ghana's burden of disease with no cost-sharing (although all enrollees except pregnant women and the poor pay a registration fee).

- Vulnerable groups—poor people, pregnant women, children, pensioners, and the elderly—are covered and exempt from premium contributions. They represent about 65 percent of enrollees.

- The NHIS is evolving as an active health purchaser. The maturing strategic purchasing function, although not yet adequately exploited, has the potential to be a force for change and modernization in service delivery.

- Consumer satisfaction levels are high: according to the 2008 Citizens Assessment Survey by the National Development Planning Commission, 92 percent of insured members are either "very satisfied" or "satisfied" with the scheme.

- Women covered by the NHIS are more likely to receive prenatal care, deliver at a hospital, have their births attended by a trained health professional, experience fewer birth complications, and experience fewer infant deaths (Mensah and others 2010; Mensah, Oppong, and Schmidt 2010).

- Between 1995 and 2009, total and public health spending increased more rapidly than GDP (nominal elasticities of 1.03 and 1.13), and private spending increased less rapidly (nominal elasticity of 0.93). Between 2004 and 2009, public health spending increased more rapidly than GDP (nominal elasticity of 1.11), total health spending increased at the same rate as GDP (nominal elasticity of 1.0), and private increased less rapidly than GDP (nominal elasticity of 0.87).

- In 2009, total spending in Ghana was slightly below or at the average level for countries with comparable levels of income (depending on the measure used), public spending was average or above average, and private spending was about average.

- Coverage under the NHIS led to better utilization by the poor of health facilities. Utilization of traditional medicines, self-medication, and forgoing of care when ill were lower for people with coverage than for people without. In the poorest quintile, utilization of essential maternal health care services was also higher among people with NHIS coverage.
- The revenue side of the NHIS appears to be stable, at least for the next three to five years, although the expenditure side faces serious difficulties (see below and chapter 4).

Weaknesses

- Between 1995 and 2009, health spending in Ghana increased less rapidly than in several African comparators and in Sub-Saharan Africa as a whole (nominal elasticity of total health spending to GDP of 1.03 in Ghana and 1.09 for Sub-Saharan Africa and a public spending elasticity of 1.13 in Ghana and 1.17 for Sub-Saharan Africa).
- Out-of-pocket spending represented 37 percent of total spending in 2009. This figure is higher than in other countries with similar levels of income and well above the 15–20 percent WHO financial protection threshold.
- In order to achieve the basic objectives of a health financing system of improving health outcomes, financial protection and consumer responsiveness in an equitable, efficient, and sustainable manner, the government and the NHIS need to better address several major challenges:
  - The NHIA is not financially viable under its current design and operational policies (for example, coverage rules, basic benefit package, provider payment and cost control, and revenue generation policies). A deficit is projected in 2010, and the reserve fund is projected to be depleted as early as 2013.
  - Rapid expansion of enrollment will not be affordable or sustainable unless cost growth is brought under control. Moreover, the HMIS of the NHIS is not capable of handling the current number of enrollees, much less an increased number.
  - Premiums, taxes, and reinsurance payments for the NHIS and to DMHISs are not actuarially determined. The premiums for informal sector workers (who make up more than 70 percent of the labor force and 29 percent of NHIS members) are low (GH¢7.2– GH¢48, depending on socioeconomic status) relative to their costs of care and regressive. Revenues from these premiums account for just 3.8 percent of total revenues.
  - The original health insurance law does not require reserves, which operational health insurance funds require in the medium to long term. Outpatient department visits per capita increased from 0.4 in 2005 to about 1.0 in 2009, and inpatient utilization increased from 22 to 58 per 1,000. Such increases may not be sustainable under current financing and provider payment arrangements.
  - Various cost-effective services are excluded, and the benefit package in general is heavily biased toward curative over preventive care. For example, family planning, which is in principle provided

by the Ministry of Health, is not part of the NHIS basic benefits package. This essential public good is underfunded, depriving the NHIS of potentially savings of $11 million in 2011 and $17 million by 2017 (Smith and Fairbank 2008).

- The extensive basic benefits package covering 95 percent of the burden of disease with no cost sharing may not be affordable or sustainable.
- Insufficient cost containment measures, including an effective gate-keeper system, are exacerbated by ineffective referral systems and misaligned incentives across insurers and provider types. As a result, much of the increase in utilization is concentrated in tertiary hospitals.
- The provider payment systems used by the NHIS are improving but have a ways to go before becoming truly effective strategic purchasing tools.
- Adverse selection and lack of enrollment of informal sector workers pervade the system, as there is no mechanism to enforce Section 31 (3) of the Health Insurance Law, which requires every person resident in Ghana (except for members of the military and police) to belong to a licensed health insurance scheme.
- Assuming the government can implement effective targeting mechanisms, large numbers of the 65 percent of enrollees who are exempt from paying premiums could afford to contribute; instead these individuals are supported by the NHIL contribution, which accounts for 61 percent of NHIS income, while the 35 percent paying members account for less than 20 percent of revenues (that is, paying members are SSNIT (6.1 percent of enrollees and 15.6 percent of revenues) and informal sector (29.4 percent of enrollees and 3.8 percent of revenues).
- Given the stringent definition of poverty, some poor and near poor are required to pay premiums, resulting in nonenrollment and reducing equity.
- Despite the numerous premium-exempt categories, neither enrollment nor the benefit incidence is pro-poor.
- Administrative/managerial efficiency is problematic. As a result of an inadequate HMIS, the system suffers from poor claims management, limited quality assurance, high administrative costs for providers and the NHIS, and incomplete information on enrollees. Other specific problems include the following:
  - The NHIA lacks common standards for certain crucial coding systems, such as procedures and pharmaceuticals.

- The NHIA does not provide adequate analytics for management of the NHIS.
- There are two competing financial systems (one provided by outsourcer STL and one provided by the Dutch engine). It is not clear whether the two systems are interfaced.
- Reimbursement delays, as well as an inadequate service accounting system, make it impossible to track patients' use of services over time.
- Tariffs are also low and accreditation of providers is incomplete.
- Targeting is weak, because of lack of coordination between the NHIA and the Ministry of Health, and enrollment is skewed toward the nonpoor.

- Specific problems areas common to many insurance entities have also emerged (see Nyonator 2010a, b, and c; Seddoh, Adjei, and Nazzar 2011):
  - difficulty identifying poor people
  - weak portability
  - unreliable eligibility authentication at provider site
  - weak control systems, which create potential for fraud
  - weak enforcement of gatekeeper system (referral system)
  - high cost of administrative inefficiencies
  - human capacity gaps
  - artificial indebtedness
  - fragmentation of claims processing centers
  - misapplication of approved tariffs
  - prescribing and dispensing of unapproved medicines
  - inefficient medical supply chain system, leading to high cost of medicines on the NHIS medicines list
  - inability to effectively monitor service utilization and cost
  - inability to gather timely data on disease patterns, hampering decision making
  - manual processing of claims, leading to delayed claims payment
  - potential for fraud by members, the DMHISs, and providers.

- Although the 2007 Public Expenditure Tracking Survey found no evidence of fund leakages, other problems are apparent:
  - There is no readily available comprehensive quantitative information on districts' finance and expenditure in Ghana.
  - There are significant delays in flows of funds (mostly from the Ministry of Finance and Economic Planning to the Ministry of Health and by districts, to and by the NHIS to districts and providers).

- ○ Funds are diverted at all levels of administrative offices.
- ○ Funds from certain sources (the out-of-pocket part of internally generated funds, funds secured to finance capital investment, and funds from national private donors) are missing.
- Demand-driven, comprehensive district health services are undersourced, as a result of the following factors:
  - ○ Development partners, the Ghana Health Service, and some parts of the NHIF increasingly ring-fence and earmark funds.
  - ○ An increasing proportion of government resources are financing statutory commitments (personnel and parts of services and investment) and ring-fenced activities.
  - ○ The costs of medicines are excessive.
  - ○ An increasing proportion of resources goes to curative services.
- Effective strategies are not in place for improving the efficiency of existing resources. The average price of medicines, for example, is two to three times the median international reference price.

Ghana's health financing system is complex, with multiple funding sources, multiple levels of government and nongovernment stakeholders, and both public and private for- and nonprofit providers. Supply-side subsidies to public facilities complicate provider payment processes, which are largely not results-based, and preclude effectively establishing a level playing field. Important data for decision making are lacking, partly as a result of an inadequate HMIS. The recent assertion by OXFAM that the NHIS covers only 18 percent of the population exemplifies the importance of better underlying information.

According to the NHIS, coverage has expanded to some 8.16 million, with further expansions planned. Vulnerable groups are covered and the benefits are extensive. The NHIS is undertaking extensive reforms in terms of its administrative structures and moving toward a much more efficient and holistic operational structure. It is seriously looking at revenue enhancements—some necessary and sensible, others politically motivated. It is working to enhance its claims-processing capabilities and improve its information base, quality, pharmaceutical management, and fraud detection.

Although the revenue base of the NHIS has been stable and gradually expanding, expenditure patterns are unsustainable. The NHIS as currently constituted in terms of its coverage rules, benefits structure, cost-sharing, exemptions policies, provider payment mechanisms, contribution requirements and expansion plans will require large increases in government contributions to be sustained and expanded, which may be difficult to justify given Ghana's macroeconomic and fiscal context (see chapter 4). Furthermore, an important adage of health insurance expansion plans is that one should not expand coverage on an inefficient and inequitable service delivery system base. For the NHIS to fulfill its promise of financial protection, significant supply-side expansions, particularly in underserved areas, will be needed, as will better targeting to ensure that enrollment is more pro-poor.

The Ministry of Health, the Ghana Health Service, and the NHIS also need to effectively deal with the plethora of delivery system and public health issues highlighted above and their deleterious effects on health outcomes. Expansions will be costly, and much of the cost will ultimately be picked up by the Ghanaian taxpayer.

Notes

1. Seddoh, Adjei, and Nazzar (2011) provide a detailed assessment of administrative and management issues affecting the NHIS.
2. There is a good deal of anecdotal evidence that informal payments are prevalent. This is an area warranting further study.

References

Akazili, J., J. Gyapong, and D. McIntyre. 2011. "Who Pays for Health Care in Ghana?" *International Journal for Equity in Health* 10 (26). http://www.equityhealthj.com/content/10/1/26.

Apoya, P., and A. Marriott. 2011. *Achieving a Shared Goal: Free Universal Health Care in Ghana*. Alliance for Reproductive Health Rights, Essential Services Platform of Ghana, Integrated Social Development Centre and Oxfam International, United Kingdom.

Appiah, E., C. Herbst, A. Soucat, and K. Saleh, eds. Forthcoming. *Towards Intervention on Human Resources for Health in Ghana: Evidence for Health Workforce Planning and Results*. Washington, DC: World Bank.

Couttolenc, B. 2012. "Decentralization and Governance in the Ghana Health Sector." World Bank, Washington, DC.

Dubbeldam, R., P. Asman, C. Cuninghame, R. McGregor, and P. K. Mensah. 2011. *Country Status Report: Health Infrastructure Management*. World Bank, Washington, DC.

Durairaj, V., S. D'Almeida, and J. Kirigia. 2010. *Ghana's Approach to Social Health Protection*. Background paper for the *World Health Report 2010*. World Health Organization, Geneva.

El Idrissi, M. 2007. *Summary of Bottleneck Analysis Used for the MBB (Mainly MDG 4, 5 and 6), 2007 and Connection with the Health System*. World Bank, Washington, DC.

Hendriks, R. 2010. *National Health Insurance Ghana*. World Bank, Washington, DC, and Ghana Ministry of Health, Accra.

IHP+ (International Health Partnerships Plus). 2010. *Joint Assessment (JANS) of Ghana's Health Sector Medium-Term Development Plan (HSMTDP) 2010–2013*. Accra.

Kutzin, J., M. Jakab, and C. Cashin. 2010. "Lessons from Health Financing Reform in Eastern Europe and the Former Soviet Union." *Health Economics, Policy and Law* 5 (2): 135–47.

Mensah, J., J. Oppong, K. Bobi-Barimah, G. Frempong, and A. Sabi. 2010. *An Evaluation of the Ghana National Health Insurance Scheme in the Context of the Health MDGs*. Global Development Network.

Mensah, J., Oppong, J. R., and C. Schmidt. 2010. "Ghana's National Health Insurance Scheme in the Context of the Health MDGs: An Empirical Evaluation Using Propensity Score Matching." *Health Economics* 19: 95–106.

National Health Insurance Authority. 2010. *Annual Report 2009*. Accra.

———. 2011. *Annual Report 2010*. Accra.

Nyonator, F. 2010a. "District Mutual Health Insurance Scheme Operations in Ghana: Key Operational Components, Quality Assurance and Challenges." PowerPoint presentation, World Bank Institute, Washington, DC.

———. 2010b. "Establishment and Governance of the National Health Insurance Scheme (NHIS) Based on District Mutual Health Insurance Schemes." PowerPoint presentation, World Bank Institute, Washington, DC.

———. 2010c. *Ghana Case Study*. World Bank Institute Health Reform Flagship Course, Washington, DC.

Saleh, Karima. Forthcoming (2012). *The Health Sector in Ghana: A Comprehensive Assessment*. Washington, DC: World Bank.

Seddoh, A., S. Adjei, and A. Nazzar. 2011. *Ghana's National Health Insurance Scheme*. Rockefeller Foundation, New York.

Sealy, S., M. Makinen, and R. Bitran. 2011. *Country Assessment of the Private Health Sector in Ghana*. World Bank, Africa Region, Washington, DC.

Seiter, A. 2011. *Country Status Report: Pharmaceutical Background Paper*. Ministry of Health and World Bank, Accra.

Smith, M., and A. Fairbank. 2008. "An Estimate of Potential Costs and Benefits of Adding Family Planning Services to the National Health Insurance Scheme in Ghana and the Impact on the Private Sector." Banking on Health Project, Accra.

WHO (World Health Organization). 2010. *World Health Report*. Geneva: WHO.

World Bank. 2007. *Ghana Public Health Expenditure Tracking System*. Africa Region, Washington, DC.

———. 2011 *Republic of Ghana: Joint Review of Public Expenditure and Financial Management*. Africa Region, Washington, DC.

World Bank and Ghana Ministry of Health. 2009. *Investing in Health in Ghana: A Review of Health Financing and the National Health Insurance Scheme*. Accra.

CHAPTER 4

Assessing the Prospects for Fiscal Space for Health in Ghana

Ghana has experienced relatively stable macroeconomic growth in recent years, creating this opportunity for more resources to be invested in social sectors. The government used the opportunity of strong economic growth to undertake rapid fiscal expansion between 2004 and 2008. Over that period, public expenditure grew from 20 percent to 24 percent of GDP (World Bank 2011a). As part of the fiscal expansion, the government increased expenditures for the health sector, particularly through the new resources dedicated to the National Health Insurance Scheme (NHIS), implemented in 2005.

The NHIS has increased both coverage and access to services. But coverage gaps remain large, and Ghana still lags behind in some important health outcomes, such as maternal mortality. In order to increase coverage, ultimately achieve universal coverage, and continue to improve health outcomes and financial protection, policy makers may need to find additional public resources and make significant improvements in the efficiency of the system over the medium to long term.

This chapter assesses possible sources of additional fiscal space, including efficiency gains that may be necessary to improve coverage and service quality within a more constrained resource envelop. It seeks to place the current discussion about increasing the coverage of the NHIS and reforming some aspects of the system, such as the premium structure and provider payment mechanisms, in a realistic macroeconomic and fiscal context.

Sources of Fiscal Space for Health

Fiscal space can be defined as "the availability of budgetary room that allows a government to provide resources for a given desired purpose without any prejudice to the sustainability of a government's financial position" (Heller 2006, p. 75). An assessment of fiscal space typically examines whether and how a government could feasibly increase its expenditure in the short to medium term in a way that is consistent with the country's macroeconomic fundamentals (Tandon and Cashin 2010).

Fiscal space for health can potentially be generated from a variety of sources, which can broadly be grouped into five categories (Heller 2006):

- conducive macroeconomic conditions, such as economic growth and increases in overall government revenue, which in turn may lead to increases in government spending for health
- the reprioritization of health within the government budget
- an increase in health sector-specific resources (through earmarked revenues, for example)
- health sector-specific grants, foreign aid, and loans
- an increase in the efficiency of existing government outlays.

Borrowing is an additional source of fiscal space. The potential for debt-financed increases in health spending can be addressed through a general assessment of macroeconomic potential and health sector-specific grants and foreign aid.

The first three options on the list usually lie outside of the domain of the health sector. They are linked to general macroeconomic policies and conditions, as well as to political economy and cross-sectoral trade-offs. Nevertheless, it is important to analyze what the implications are for the health sector of changes in the general macroeconomic and political environment within which it operates.

Fiscal space for health can be visualized using a spider plot (figure 4.1). The five axes represent each possible source of increased fiscal space for health; the "spokes" represent hypothetical examples of the predicted increases along each axis in terms of percentage increases in real government health spending over any base year.

Figure 4.1   Dimensions of Fiscal Space for Health

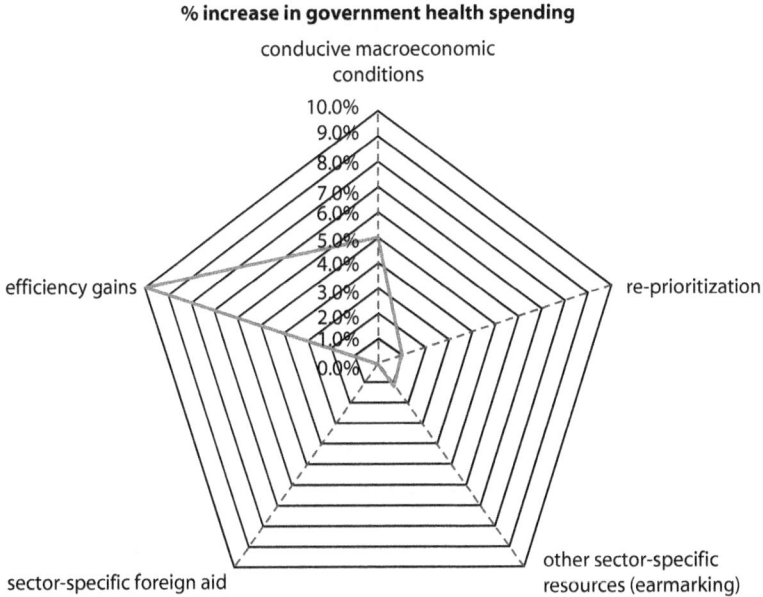

% increase in government health spending

Source: Tandon and Cashin 2010.
Note: The grey line shows the potential percentage increase in government health spending in each of the five categories. Points close to the center (such as sector-specific foreign aid) indicate little potential for increase in that category; points farther from the center (such as efficiency gains) indicate more potential for increase. The area bounded by the rules indicates the potential for increasing fiscal space for health from all sources.

Does Ghana Need Additional Fiscal Space for Health?

The potential need for additional fiscal space for health in Ghana is driven by the government's commitment to strengthen the NHIS and substantially expand its coverage to include more individuals from poor and vulnerable groups as well as the remaining uninsured population. The NHIS has made significant achievements since it was launched. The rapid growth in utilization and total claims has posed challenges for cost containment and sustainability, however. The average annual cost of total claims per member more than doubled between 2007 and 2009 (NHIA 2010). Moreover, it may be more costly to expand coverage to more poor and vulnerable households. The current subsidy level for exempt groups and the premiums for self-employed and informal sector members are not actuarially determined. As the uncovered population may not be able to afford an actuarially fair premium, the government subsidy contribution may need to increase if coverage is to grow, which will require additional fiscal contributions.

On the service delivery side, significant investment may be needed to upgrade and expand the supply network and make services available in underserved areas to meet the commitments in the NHIS benefit package. The Ministry of Health's costing of its medium-term development plan estimates that GH¢1.8–GH¢13.4 million in investment funds will be needed between 2010 and 2013 to upgrade service delivery, expand the network of community-based health planning and services compounds to extend the reach of primary care, and provide preserve training for an adequate number of health professionals.

How Can Ghana Increase Its Fiscal Space for Health?

This section provides a systematic assessment of the potential for increasing fiscal space for health in Ghana from each of the five main sources: conducive macroeconomic conditions, reprioritization of health, health-sector specific sources, foreign aid, and efficiency. The analysis relies on the most recent macroeconomic and fiscal data for Ghana from multiple sources, particularly the International Monetary Fund (IMF 2011a, 2011b), official government statistics, and the 2011 World Bank Public Expenditure Review (World Bank 2011a). Official data were supplemented by a two-week field visit to Ghana to interview key policymakers and stakeholders and by an in-depth review of the government's macroeconomic, fiscal, and health sector–specific policies and strategies and assessments of their implementation.

Conducive Macroeconomic Conditions

Conducive macroeconomic conditions—such as sustained economic growth, improvements in revenue generation, and low levels of fiscal deficits and debt—are important sources of new fiscal space for any sector. High levels of economic growth can lead to increases in fiscal space for health even if the share of GDP devoted to government spending on health remains unchanged. If a country has low fiscal deficits and in general keeps its debt under control, deficit financing is another way to generate new fiscal resources in the short run. However, deficit financing is not sustainable in the long-run.

Unchecked expansionary policies in 2004–08 contributed new resources to the health sector but also led to a near macroeconomic crisis. The stabilization program undertaken by the government since 2009 has had rapid effects on the overall health of the economy in Ghana, but the gains remain fragile and the job of clearing arrears and strengthening overall public financial management is far from over.

The current macroeconomic landscape in Ghana warrants cautious optimism in the near to medium term.[1] The economy is projected to expand by more than 14 percent in 2011, evenly divided between growth of the nonoil economy and the start of oil production (IMF 2011a and b). Although oil production will generate a spike in growth over the next year or two, the increase is not expected to be sustained, with projected growth rates returning to about 6 percent a year starting in 2013 (figure 4.2). The prospects for economic growth in Ghana therefore remain modest but steady, with the potential to generate some limited additional fiscal space for health over the next three to five years.

From historical trends, economic growth in Ghana can be expected to translate at least proportionally into increased government health expenditure. Total health expenditure, as well as the government's share of total health expenditure, generally increase with national income in most countries. The responsiveness, or "elasticity," of government health

Figure 4.2   Actual and Projected Real Annual GDP Growth in Ghana, 1998–2015

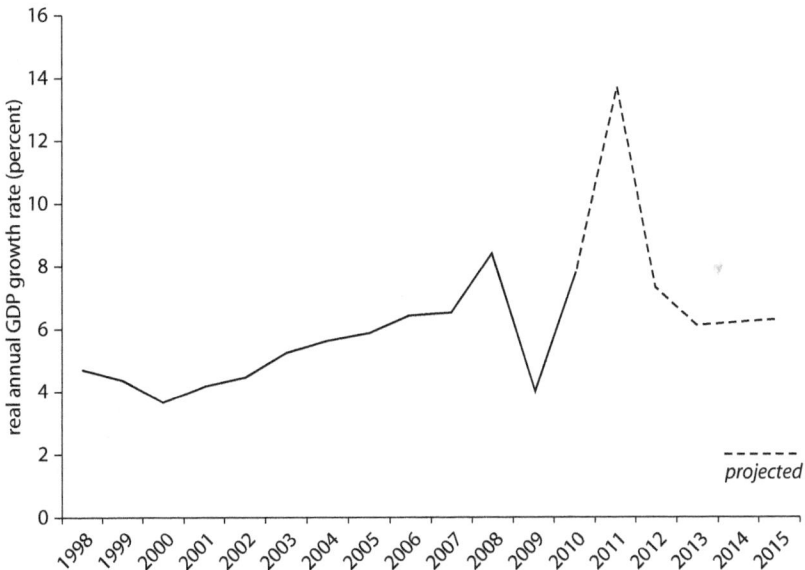

expenditure with respect to GDP gives an indication of whether favorable macroeconomic conditions can be expected to translate into more public expenditure on health. The nominal elasticity of government spending to GDP is estimated to be about 1.16 across all low-income countries (implying that on average, a 1 percent rise in income leads to a 1.16 percent rise in government health spending) (Tandon and Cashin 2010). For Sub-Saharan Africa, the elasticity was estimated to be 1.17 for the period 1995–2009. The responsiveness of government spending was slightly lower in Ghana (1.13).

If economic growth reaches and sustains at least the modest projected levels and government health expenditure increases at least proportionally, consistent with Ghana's total health expenditure experience over 1995–2009, cumulative nominal government health expenditure could increase by 55 percent by 2015 (table 4.1). Adjusting for inflation, however, real government health expenditure would actually decrease by 13 percent. The contraction in real government health expenditure is more severe if oil revenue is excluded from GDP growth, reaching almost a 20 percent decline.

Under a more optimistic scenario, in which government health spending responds to GDP growth at a level consistent with the Sub-Saharan average elasticity of 1.17, nominal government health expenditure would increase by 75 percent. Real expenditure would still decline, by about 1 percent.

Economic growth translates into fiscal space only if it generates additional government revenue. Although Ghana has made recent progress toward more effective revenue generation, tax revenue reached only 15 percent of GDP in 2010, falling well below the average of 20 percent of GDP for lower middle-income countries (World Bank estimates).

The rebasing of Ghana's GDP in November 2010 exposed the weakness in Ghana's revenue collection efforts. Previous GDP estimates showed revenue collection rates of more than 20 percent of GDP, which made revenue collection a low priority for new public finance measures. When the GDP was rebased, however, the steep drop in the revenue/GPD ratio highlighted the need for a comprehensive review of collection procedures and processes (Ghana Revenue Authority 2011). There seems to be some scope for increasing fiscal space by improving revenue collection in Ghana. The government is committed to taking the necessary steps to bring revenue collection closer to international standards.

Ghana is pursuing a number of measures to improve revenue collection. In 2010 it established an integrated revenue authority, the Ghana

Table 4.1 Estimated Additional Fiscal Space for Health in Ghana from Economic Growth, 2010–15

(dollars, except where otherwise indicated)

	2010	2011	2012	2013	2014	2015
Oil revenue as projected; elasticity of government health expenditure to GDP = 1.000						
Projected nominal government health expenditure	837,982,600	941,054,460	1,020,103,034	1,083,349,423	1,151,600,436	1,220,696,462
Projected real estimated health expenditure[a]	450,298,408	454,577,694	453,527,666	443,662,852	430,162,005	418,303,892
Real growth rate (percent)		1.0	−0.2	−2.2	−3.0	−2.8
Nominal cumulative growth 2009–15 (percent)	54.5					
Real cumulative growth 2009–15 (percent)	−13.6					
Oil revenue excluded; elasticity of government health expenditure to GDP = 1.000						
Projected nominal government health expenditure	830,907,700	884,916,701	943,321,203	1,005,580,402	1,072,954,289	1,144,842,226
Projected real estimated health expenditure[a]	446,496,639	427,460,269	419,391,227	411,814,193	400,784,989	392,310,434
Real growth rate (percent)		−4.3	−1.9	−1.8	−2.7	−2.1
Nominal cumulative growth 2009–15 (percent)	45.6					
Real cumulative growth 2009–15 (percent)	−18.6					

(continued next page)

Table 4.1 *(continued)*

	2010	2011	2012	2013	2014	2015
Oil revenue as projected; elasticity of government health expenditure to GDP = 1.172						
Projected nominal government health expenditure	846,906,407	968,993,047	1,064,388,475	1,141,731,199	1,226,032,064	1,312,246,638
Projected real estimated health expenditure[a]	455,093,706	468,073,468	473,216,533	467,571,874	457,964,754	449,675,979
Real growth rate (percent)	–5.6	2.9	1.1	–1.2	–2.1	–1.8
Nominal cumulative growth 2009–15 (percent)	66.9					
Real cumulative growth 2009–15 (percent)	–6.7					
Oil revenue excluded; elasticity of government health expenditure to GDP = 1.172						
Projected nominal government health expenditure	846,906,407	911,423,737	981,924,186	1,057,877,986	1,140,946,797	1,230,538,503
Projected real estimated health expenditure[a]	455,093,706	440,264,531	436,553,730	433,231,563	426,182,508	421,676,527
Real growth rate (percent)	–5.6	–3.3	–0.8	–0.8	–1.6	–1.1
Nominal cumulative growth 2009–15 (percent)	56.5					
Real cumulative growth 2009–15 (percent)	–12.5					

Source: Authors, based on World Bank estimates.
a. Deflated by GDP deflator with 2006 as the base year.

Revenue Authority. Other measures include reviewing the policy of using tax waivers and exemptions as incentives for attracting foreign direct investment; introducing new taxes, such as a communications service tax; and tightening tax enforcement (IMF 2011a, 2011b). Contrary to widespread perceptions, the government does not expect oil production to be a major driver of new revenue, with projected tax revenue from upstream petroleum amounting to only 4.3 percent of total tax revenue (Ghana Revenue Authority 2011). Furthermore, the Petroleum Revenue Management Act (Act 815) stipulates that 30 percent of petroleum revenue is to be saved in two special funds; only 70 percent will be made available for the general budget.

Significant increases in government revenue are expected from the new revenue collection efficiency measures recently put in place and planned for the near future. With all of these efforts starting immediately, the Ghana Revenue Authority expects a 27 percent growth in revenue for 2011, an estimate supported by World Bank and IMF projections (figure 4.3). These projections may appear overly optimistic given the

Figure 4.3   Actual and Projected Tax Collection in Ghana, 2008–15

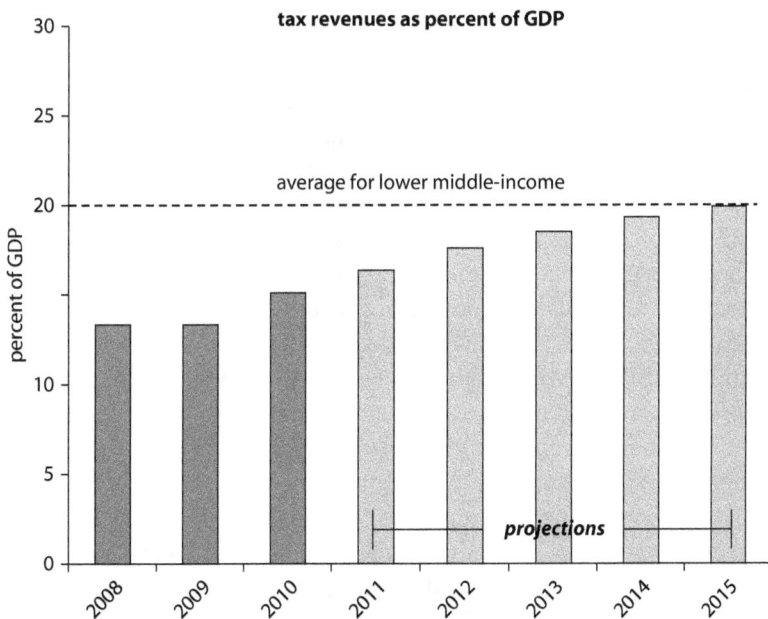

Source: World Bank and IMF estimates.

challenges that remain for revenue generation in Ghana, such as the slow pace of automation of the functions of the revenue authorities and the large share of informal economic activity. In fact, the IMF's targets for revenue collection were met or exceeded, because of higher customs collections of value added taxes and trade taxes after tax administration was strengthened (IMF 2011a, 2011b).

If these projections continue to be met, the additional revenue that will be generated over the next five years will be an important, possibly one of the most important, sources of new fiscal space for health, particularly when compounded by the increased revenue that is expected from economic growth (table 4.2). Assuming that the share of new government revenue that is allocated to the health sector stays at least constant, real government health expenditure could increase by more than 27 percent. Of that, 11–32 percent of the increase is directly attributable to improved revenue collection (figure 4.4). If government health spending increases slightly more than proportionally to revenue, real government health expenditure could increase by 45 percent, with 12–36 percent directly attributable to improved revenue collection.

Increased fiscal resources for health also can be generated by borrowing. Because Ghana only recently began getting its economy back into balance after a debt-fueled expansionary period from 2004 to 2008, any large-scale debt-financed investment strategies or even deficit-financed countercyclical fiscal expansion is unlikely, however (UNDP 2011). After peaking at 40 percent in 2010, Ghana's public debt is predicted to gradually decline for the next several years. The fiscal deficit is projected to be brought under control by 2014. In order to meet these important elements of its macroeconomic and fiscal stabilization plans, the government is unlikely to consider large-scale debt-financed fiscal expansion.

The prospects for increasing fiscal space for health in Ghana through economic growth and better mobilization of government revenues could be significant, at least over the next five years. Even under the conservative assumption that economic growth levels off at a modest 6–7 percent a year, real government health expenditure could increase by up to 45 percent by 2015 from the starting point in 2009. This new fiscal space will be possible, however, only if enhanced revenue collection efforts are successful and Ghana achieves a collection rate of 20 percent of GDP by 2015.

Figure 4.5 shows two possible scenarios for changes in real government expenditure between 2009 and 2015. The base scenario includes no improvement in revenue collection and government health expenditure responding proportionally to increases in GDP and government revenue.

Table 4.2 Estimated Additional Fiscal Space for Health in Ghana from Improved Revenue Collection, 2010–15

(dollars, except where otherwise indicated)

	2010	2011	2012	2013	2014	2015
Oil revenue as projected; elasticity of government health expenditure to GDP = 1.000						
Projected nominal government health expenditure	937,031,200	1,136,618,846	1,327,570,812	1,477,586,313	1,637,165,635	1,794,333,536
Projected real estimated health expenditure[a]	503,523,173	549,045,348	590,224,783	605,114,235	611,537,153	614,875,790
Real growth rate (percent)	4.5	9.0	7.5	2.5	1.1	0.5
Share attributable to improved revenue collection (percent)	11.3	16.9	23.6	27.2	30.2	32.3
Nominal cumulative growth 2009–15 (percent)	128.0					
Real cumulative growth 2009–15–(percent)	27.6					
Oil revenue excluded; elasticity of government health expenditure to GDP = 1.000						
Projected nominal government health expenditure	864,710,000	951,181,000	1,046,299,100	1,150,929,010	1,266,021,911	1,392,624,102
Projected real estimated health expenditure[a]	464,660,646	459,469,333	465,174,176	471,338,643	472,902,325	477,219,440
Real growth rate (percent)	-3.6	-1.1	1.2	1.3	0.3	0.9
Share attributable to improved revenue collection (percent)	3.9	7.0	9.8	12.6	15.2	17.8
Nominal cumulative growth 2009–15 (percent)	77.0					
Real cumulative growth 2009–15 (percent)	-1.0					
Oil revenue as projected; elasticity of government health expenditure to GDP = 1.172						
Projected nominal government health expenditure	962,991,366	1,203,388,679	1,440,331,097	1,631,082,786	1,837,538,720	2,044,283,877
Projected real estimated health expenditure[a]	517,473,131	581,298,611	640,356,884	667,975,470	686,383,329	700,527,878
Real growth rate (percent)	7.4	12.3	10.2	4.3	2.8	2.1
Share attributable to improved revenue collection (percent)	12.1	19.5	26.1	30.0	33.3	35.8
Nominal cumulative growth 2009–15 (percent)	160.0					
Real cumulative growth 2009–15 (percent)	45.4					
Oil revenue excluded; elasticity of government health expenditure to GDP = 1.172						
Projected nominal government health expenditure	878,230,920	981,159,584	1,096,151,487	1,224,620,441	1,368,145,957	1,504,960,553
Projected real estimated health expenditure[a]	471,926,249	473,950,531	487,338,052	501,517,410	511,049,136	515,714,493
Real growth rate (percent)	-2.1	0.4	2.8	2.9	1.9	0.9
Share attributable to improved revenue collection (percent)	3.6	7.1	10.4	13.6	16.6	18.2
Nominal cumulative growth 2009–15 (percent)	91.0					
Real cumulative growth 2009–15 (percent)	7.0					

Source: Authors, based on World Bank estimates.

a. Deflated by GDP deflator with 2006 as the base year.

Figure 4.4   Actual and Projected Additional Fiscal Space for Health in Ghana as a Result of Economic Growth and Improved Revenue Collection, 2009–15

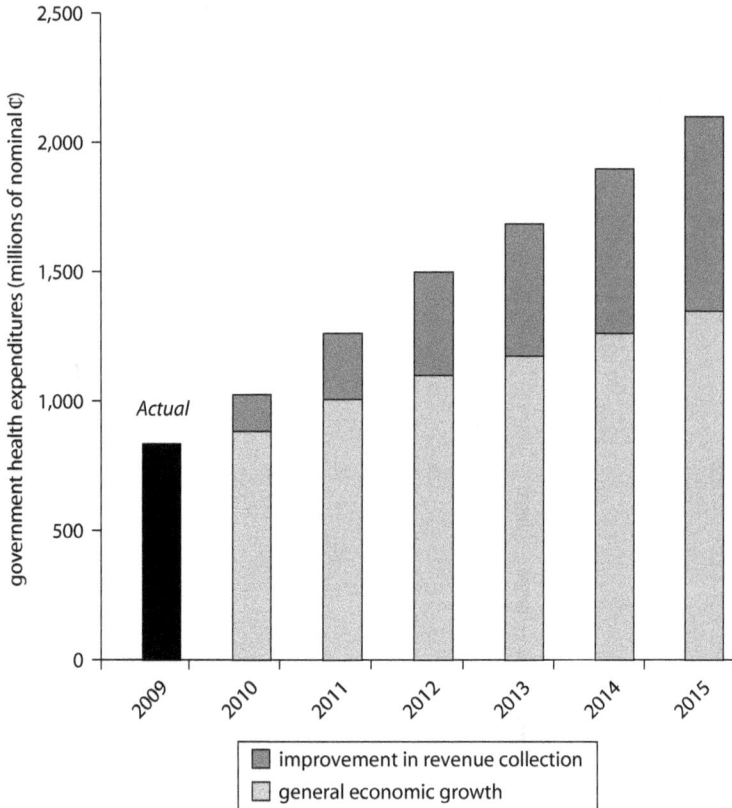

Source: Authors, based on World Bank estimates.

In the optimistic scenario, new revenue collection efforts are successful, and government health spending responds to GDP with an elasticity that is consistent with the average for Sub-Saharan Africa (1.17). Under the base scenario, real government health spending declines 13 percent; under the optimistic scenario, real government health expenditure rises by as much as 45 percent.

Reprioritization of Health

There may be scope for raising the share of overall government spending devoted to health, if revenue effort increases and the government continues its expansion of NHIS, particularly if it focuses on enrolling more

**Figure 4.5   Projected Change in Government Health Spending 2009–15 Under
Base and Optimistic Scenarios**

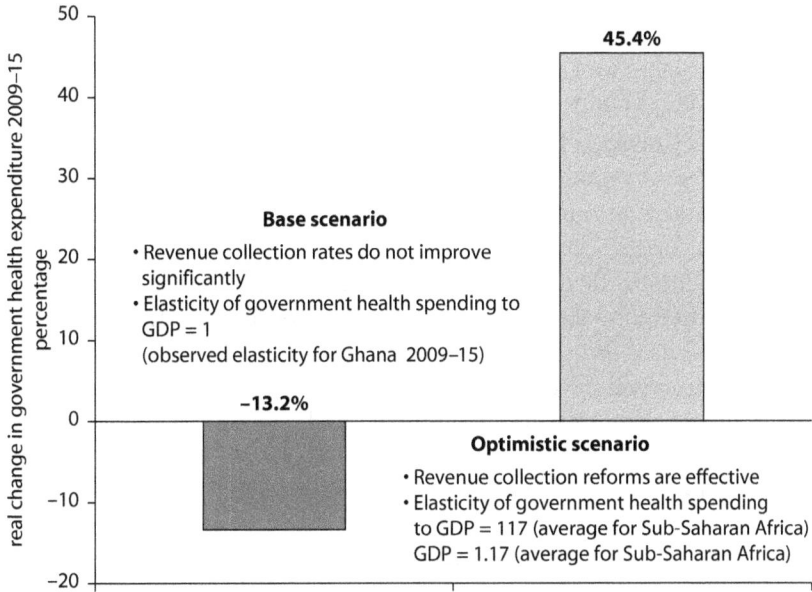

Base scenario
- Revenue collection rates do not improve
  significantly
- Elasticity of government health spending to
  GDP = 1
  (observed elasticity for Ghana 2009–15)

Optimistic scenario
- Revenue collection reforms are effective
- Elasticity of government health spending
  to GDP = 117 (average for Sub-Saharan Africa)
  GDP = 1.17 (average for Sub-Saharan Africa)

Source: Authors, based on World Bank estimates.

poor people. Introduction of the NHIS drove a major increase in budget
resources for the health sector, whose budget increased from GH¢120
million in 2004 to GH¢507 million in 2008. Expenditure by the National
Health Insurance Fund (NHIF) added GH¢330 million to the budget in
2009. Although budgetary funds for the health sector are increasing,
actual transfers to the NHIF have been far below budgeted amounts
(NHIA 2010), and the share of the total budget allocated to health has
remained relatively stagnant.

The share of the government budget allocated to health has remained
at about 12–13 percent in recent years—below the 15 percent Abuja
target set by African heads of state in 2001 at the African Union sum-
mit in Nigeria. It is not clear, however, that Ghana's budget share for
health can be considered low. The Abuja target is not universally
accepted (Health Systems 20/20 2008), and, as shown in chapter 2,
other countries in Sub-Saharan African region spend a much smaller
share of their budget on health. Kenya, for example, allocated 7.1 percent
of its budget to health in 2008, and Nigeria allocated only 6.5 percent
(World Bank 2011b).

It is unlikely that Ghana's budget share for health will increase significantly over the medium term. The budget structure in Ghana allows little room for resource reallocation. Ghana's large public sector wage bill consumes almost 60 percent of total government revenues (World Bank 2011a). In addition, four statutory funds (the National Health Insurance Fund, the Road Fund, the Ghana Education Trust Fund, and the District Assemblies Common Fund), as well as other obligatory demands on government resources, such as debt servicing, take up a significant portion of the government resource envelope. The implementation of the new wage policy (the Single Spine Salary Structure) is likely to absorb much of any limited additional flexible resources that may be available in the medium term. Furthermore, the government priorities outlined in the 2011 budget and the medium-term development framework identify job creation and infrastructural development as priorities. Plans for major investment in several priority areas—agriculture, oil and gas, natural resources, and road and rail transport (Government of Ghana 2010)—will put additional demands on the budget (World Bank 2011a).

Health Sector–Specific Resources

Health sector–specific resources—such as earmarked taxation or the introduction of mandatory health insurance—can provide additional fiscal space for the sector. Earmarking can involve dedicating an entire tax to fund a particular program (for example, a dedicated payroll tax earmarked for social health insurance) or setting aside a fixed portion of a particular tax to fund the program (for example, a fixed proportion of general tax revenues allocated to the health budget). User fees or direct out-of-pocket payments to government facilities can also provide additional fiscal space.

Resources earmarked for the National Health Insurance Scheme. Ghana has already introduced an earmarked tax for health to fund the NHIS. The "health insurance levy" earmarks 2.5 percent of the VAT for the NHIS. In addition, 2.5 percentage points of the 18.5 percent contribution to the Social Security and National Insurance Trust (SSNIT) by formal (public and private) sector workers is earmarked for the NHIS. Investment income, premiums paid by nonexempt individuals, and grants also fund the NHIS (table 4.3).

According to recent projections, the resources available to the NHIS from combined sources will remain stable and continue to grow at modest rates. The volume of funds available to the NHIA from the 2.5 percent health insurance levy is expected to increase by about 20 percent a year

Table 4.3   Revenues of the National Health Insurance Authority, by Source, 2005–09

(dollars)

Source	2005	2006	2007	2008	2009
Value Added Tax					
(VAT)	1,596,219	117,553,900	166,659,642	203,392,292	262,157,158
Social Security and National Insurance Trust					
(SSNIT)	264,870	40,969,800	55,016,488	55,801,398	67,301,972
Grants	17,326			16,864,000	10,558,984
Investment income	7,817	6,803,900	27,543,028	36,148,113	75,640,895
Premiums				18,092,732	
Other	165		37,733	474,423	1,020,299
Total	1,886,397	165,354,900	249,256,891	330,772,958	416,679,308

Source: Authors, based on NHIA data.

over the next three years. Revenue from SSNIT contributions is also expected to grow substantially. The number of SSNIT contributors is directly related to the growth of Ghana's economy and the degree of formal sector inclusion in the labor market. As the economy is projected to grow at a strong pace for the next several years, the revenue for NHIS coming from SSNIT is projected to increase by almost 60 percent over the 2009 level by 2012 (World Bank estimates).

There has been a trend toward greater diversification of funding sources for the NHIS (figure 4.6). Whereas the health insurance levy contributed more than 70 percent of the total revenues of the NHIA in 2006, the share was only slightly more than 60 percent in 2009. The share contributed by SSNIT also declined, from a high of 24.8 percent in 2006 to 15.5 percent in 2009. A large increase in the importance of investment income has made up most of the difference.

The role of premiums paid by people who are self-employed or work in the informal sector has been difficult to assess. As these premiums are paid directly to the district mutual schemes, they have not been fully reflected in the accounting reports of the NHIA. Although an effort is being made to account for this revenue source, the figures currently reported are likely to be an underestimate.

Most people covered by the NHIS are exempt from paying premiums. About 60 percent fall into a group that is exempt from paying premiums (the poor, SSNIT pensioners, children under 18, people 70 and over, and

Figure 4.6   Sources of Revenue of the National Health Insurance Authority, 2005–09

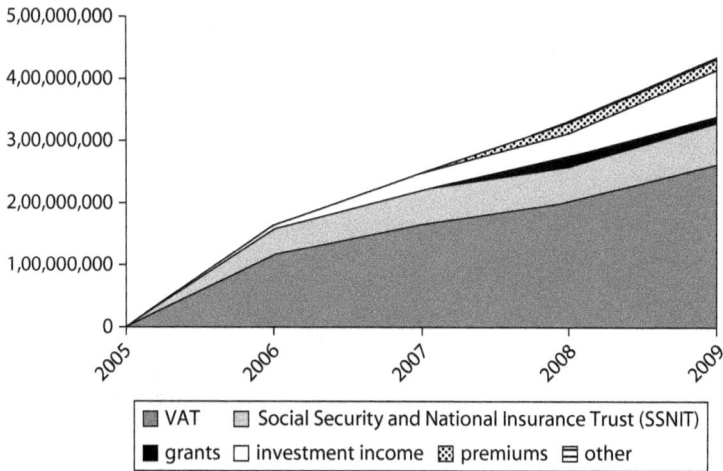

Source: Authors, based on NHIA data.

pregnant women); another 6 percent contribute through SSNIT rather than paying premiums. Annual premiums range from GH₵7.20–GH₵48, although it is not clear what share of enrollees pay the different premium levels or whether in practice there is any means testing. Identifying indigent enrollees has been left to the district schemes, which seem to grant exemptions ad hoc. There is a movement toward unifying means-tested targeting criteria through the Livelihood Empowerment Against Poverty (LEAP), but it is not clear whether using the LEAP criteria would increase or decrease the number and share of individuals eligible for premium exemption under the NHIS.

Investment income has been an important revenue source for the NHIS, but it depends on the size of the reserve fund. Investment income has grown significantly since the NHIF was established. Growth rates from year to year range from a low of 30 percent in 2007 to a high of 300 percent in 2006. In 2009, investment income doubled over the previous year. Investment income is an important revenue source and one that will become threatened if the NHIA continues to draw on the reserve fund to cover deficits.

Grants typically contribute less than 5 percent of the total revenue of the NHIS. As Ghana is moving toward middle-income status, it is unlikely that grants in general, and grants for the NHIS in particular, will increase significantly over the next three to five years.

Other earmarked taxes. Increasing taxes specifically on goods that adversely affect health, notably tobacco and alcohol, can generate revenue that can be earmarked for the health sector. "Sin taxes" can be justified by the externalities associated with the goods on which they are imposed. Taxation to reduce consumption of such "bads" is considered beneficial not only from a public health perspective but also from an economic perspective. Even if they are not earmarked for health, higher taxes can discourage consumption and reduce illness and accidents (in the case of alcohol), possibly reducing demand for health services, which benefits all of society. Australia, the Republic of Korea, and the United States have successfully implemented earmarked taxes on tobacco and used the revenues for public health purposes (Tandon and Cashin 2010).

Ghana's tobacco control policy is beginning to evolve, and there may be scope (albeit limited) for including earmarked taxes on tobacco products as a strategic part of this policy, as well as a source of funds for the health sector. Ghana is a member of the WHO Framework Convention on Tobacco Control, an evidence-based treaty developed in response to the globalization of the tobacco epidemic (WHO 2005). Some new tobacco control measures have been put in place since Ghana ratified the framework (Owusu-Dabo and others 2010). In particular, taxes on tobacco have increased, although the tax rate remains low by international standards at about 31 percent of the retail price (MOH 2010). The needs assessment carried out by the Ministry of Health for compliance with the Framework Convention on Tobacco Control noted that both the Ministry of Finance and Economic Planning and the Parliamentary Health Committee expressed some interest in at least examining international experience with earmarked taxation for tobacco to fund tobacco control and other public health activities.

Internally generated funds. Four sources fund public health facilities in Ghana:

- the Ministry of Health budget (for salaries, some other recurrent costs, and investment)
- payments for services delivered under the NHIS
- out-of-pocket ("cash and carry") payments by individuals not covered by the NHIS or using services not included in the benefits package

- other sources, such as private insurance payments or grants from international agencies or local government.

The last three sources are considered "internally generated funds." They are treated as supplemental income to the facilities to cover the recurrent costs associated with service delivery. Internally generated funds have increased in importance for public facilities in Ghana, rising from just under 14 percent of revenue in 2005 to 23 percent in 2009. Although the data do not permit disaggregation, much of that increase is accounted for by the NHIS. Nonetheless, out-of-pocket payments continue to be widespread.

In their current form, out-of-pocket payments are likely to be inequitable and are not likely to improve the efficiency of service utilization. The severe political backlash against "cash and carry" has prevented any discussion of copayments in the NHIS. The amount of out-of-pocket funding for health care remains large in Ghana, however; if these private payments could be harnessed under the NHIS, they could be used more effectively. In the context of a well-defined benefits package with targeted exemptions, imposition of copayments for some covered services by some populations able to pay may be able to achieve multiple objectives.

Health Sector–Specific Grants and Foreign Aid

Donor assistance contributed more than 25 percent of total government health spending in 2009 (MOH 2009). These resources are mostly inflexible and therefore of less value to the government than other sources of fiscal space. More than 60 percent of donor funding is earmarked for particular programs. The more flexible sector budget support, which can be applied to government health priorities, makes up only about 30 percent of donor funding.

Donor support for the health sector in Ghana is projected to decline starting in 2011. Although the projections shown in figure 4.7 are likely to underestimate funding, donor funding should not be considered a reliable source of future fiscal space for health in Ghana. Because it recently achieved lower-middle income status, Ghana will face reduced access to concessional lending and grants. A report by the United Nations Development Programme (UNDP 2011) suggests that Ghana would benefit from improving its credit rating and devising a clear exit strategy from aid.

Figure 4.7   Actual and Projected Donor Contributions to Ghana's Health Sector, 2008–13

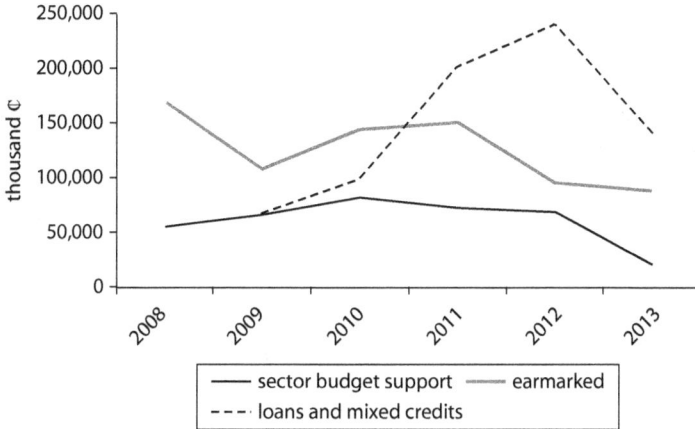

Source: Authors, based on Ministry of Health data.
Note: Figures for 2008–10 are actual; figures for 2011–13 are projections.

Potential Efficiency Gains

Fiscal space can also be realized through efficiency gains—producing more output, coverage, or quality from the same level of health expenditure. In some cases, high levels of inefficiency limit the absorptive capacity of additional resources; addressing inefficiency may be considered a precondition for bringing significant additional resources into the system. Interventions aimed at improving the technical and allocative efficiency of health spending include using cost-effectiveness criteria to inform resource allocations, reducing leakages in interfiscal transfers, and addressing absenteeism (Tandon and Cashin 2010).

Several structural inefficiencies in Ghana's health system, as well as in the operations of the NHIS, likely consume a large share of resources in the system. Addressing these inefficiencies would not only free up additional fiscal space already in the system, it would also increase the absorptive capacity for future resources. A few of the most serious inefficiencies in Ghana's health system are identified in the subsections that follow.

Poorly planned investment in hospital infrastructure. NHIS provider payment and certification procedures have important impacts on access, supply, quality, and the efficiency of the service delivery infrastructure. In addition to direct "insurance" reimbursements to Ministry of Health facilities, which accounted for 18 percent of ministry revenues and 71 percent of NHIS expenditures in 2009 (NHIA 2010), there are also direct payments from the NHIS to fund the Ministry of Health and the Ghana Health Service. These payments accounted for 14 percent of ministry revenues and 9 percent of NHIS expenditures in 2009. The purpose and appropriateness of these payments need to be assessed. Should a national health insurance organization be supporting a significant share of the Ministry of Health budget beyond reimbursement for services? Do these payments represent a simple substitution of earmarked funds for general budget funds to give the Ministry of Finance and Economic Planning additional flexibility? If these are legitimate payments for covered services to NHIS beneficiaries, it is unclear why all of the payments are not being made directly to the facilities.

Low productivity and high administrative costs of health facilities. Although systematic data are not available, a recent public expenditure review found that emoluments and administrative costs make up an "exceptionally large" share of health facility expenditure and that productivity is low. Although health worker salaries have increased significantly— health staff salaries are now 21 percent higher than salaries in other service sectors—there is no performance-based management or other forms of accountability for health facility staff (World Bank 2011a).

Orientation toward curative rather than primary and preventive care. Inadequate access to basic primary care services at the local level can create inefficiency through inappropriate bypassing of primary care for higher-level facilities or delaying of treatment until health conditions worsen (and become more expensive to treat). Ghana has committed to addressing the problems of access to basic primary care services in some areas of the country, which could be a source of future efficiency gains. Expanding the community-based health program and services (CHPS) is the main strategy for strengthening primary care service delivery (MOH 2011). CHPS zones include a resident community health nurse in a resourced community health post. Significant investment will be needed up front, however, to achieve the objective of establishing CHPS zones in at least 80 percent of the 16,000 local government units.

The NHIS benefit package is also weighted toward curative rather than primary and preventive care. There are few incentives in the system for either providers or patients to expand access to and use of preventive care. Paying for preventive services (such as screening for chronic diseases), family planning, and possibly even nonmedical prevention (such as insecticide-treated nets for malaria) could generate savings by reducing demand for more expensive services and medications (Smith and

Fairbank 2008). Furthermore, payment systems such as capitation, which encourage and reward prevention and keep the enrolled population healthy, may generate both immediate savings (by limiting total expenditure) and a structural shift in expenditure patterns over the longer term.

Eligibility for subsidy. The NHIS is a highly subsidized system; subsidies to individuals who are able to pay for premiums can be considered a source of inefficiency in the use of public resources. Currently, more than 65 percent of enrollees are in groups that are exempt from premiums. Enrollees under the age of 18 and over the age of 69 account for about 80 percent of all exempt individuals. Some estimates suggest that 46 percent of these individuals are in the top two wealth quintiles of the population.[2] Targeting the government subsidy for the NHIS premium to the truly indigent and requiring means-tested contributions from others would free up government resources to cover more of the poor.

NHIS provider payment systems. The NHIS pays hospitals and outpatient departments a flat rate for each treated case, depending on the diagnosis (Ghana Diagnostics Related Group [G-DRG]). Although the G-DRG payment system is an improvement over the previous traditional fee-for-service payment system, it includes no cap on claims, leaving payment to providers open ended. Utilization and total claims have continued to increase at unsustainable rates, with no mechanism to ensure that funding is allocated in the most cost-effective way. Several easily corrected aspects of the design of the G-DRG payment system such as the "maximum" payment of three visits for complicated malaria, which has evolved into a minimum—also contribute to inefficiency and the overuse of services.

A pilot is being planned in the Ashanti region to test capitated payment for primary care; discussions continue about better enforcement of a gatekeeping system. It is critical, however, for the NHIS to develop a comprehensive purchasing and provider payment strategy that creates incentives across the continuum of care to improve quality and use services in a cost-effective way.

Payment for medications. Pharmaceuticals account for about half of NHIS spending, and the NHIS accounts for about 44 percent of total pharmaceutical spending (the complex range of pharmaceutical issues are discussed in the Country Status Report [Saleh forthcoming] and a background paper on pharmaceuticals [Seiter 2011]). Major issues concern not just prices and spending but quality, prescribing patterns, fraud and abuse, and, most critically, patient health outcomes. Chapter 5 discusses possible savings from changes in pharmaceutical polices.

Operational inefficiencies. Delays in claims processing have been a major source of inefficiency within the NHIS. Until recently, the NHIS could have a backlog of several months of unprocessed claims. Delays in payments to providers create enormous inefficiencies, depriving providers of a reliable flow of funds with which to operate their facilities. Because of delays in payment, providers may run out of essential supplies and medicines or be forced to buy them on credit or charge patients directly. Long payment delays also dilute the incentives of provider payment systems and create inefficiencies for the NHIS.

It has been difficult to monitor expenditure flows and get a clear picture of the actual costs of operating the system. Progress has been made to reduce delays for claims processed through the national NHIS claims processing unit. As claims processing is further centralized, it will be a challenge to continue to automate and streamline processing to maintain the reduced turn-around times. Several potential efficiency gains, such as expanding CHPS zones and further automating NHIS claims processing, will require upfront investment in order to realize future savings.

Conclusions

Ghana has modest prospects for creating additional fiscal space for health over the next three to five years, but real growth in resources for the health sector depends to a certain extent on oil revenue and the ability of the government to significantly improve its revenue collection efforts as planned. Major efficiency gains are needed to generate additional fiscal space for health and improve the absorptive capacity for existing and new resources flowing into the system. Under any scenario, additional fiscal space from macroeconomic growth and improved revenue collection will begin to slow after 2013 based on current economic projections.

Earmarked funding sources will provide a high degree of stability in revenues into the foreseeable future. Revenue for the NHIS will continue to grow robustly. The revenue will not be sufficient to sustain and expand the NHIS, however, under current expenditure patterns. If the structural inefficiencies in the NHIS and the health service delivery system are not addressed, the NHIS is projected to become insolvent as early as 2013. It is difficult to argue for bringing additional resources into an inefficient system without accompanying structural and operational changes.

Chapter 5 presents a comprehensive set of reform options. Adopting reforms that address both the revenue and expenditure sides could make the NHIS viable and sustainable beyond the short term.

Notes

1. The degree to which Ghana's economy now lies on a more solid foundation is not clear. The Poverty Reduction Support Credit report of December 2010 and the United Nations Development Programme's *Leveraging Fiscal Space for Human Development in Ghana* of January 2011 treat recent gains as tenuous; the Joint Review of Public Expenditure and Management (World Bank 2011a) takes a slightly more optimistic tone. The stabilization measures have been in place for only two years, however; many of the more optimistic assessments are based on planned rather than institutionalized policy changes. It therefore seems prudent to consider recent gains as fragile, with long-term stability still in question.

2. Under current arrangements, children 18 and under are covered if both parents are covered by the NHIS. A ministerial decree was issued delinking children's eligibility from their parents' eligibility; legislation is still pending to drop the parent enrollment requirement.

References

Ghana Revenue Authority. 2011. Statement by Commissioner-General, GRA, Mr. George Blankson at a Media Briefing on Monday 31st January 2011. http://www.gra.gov.gh/index.php?option=com_contentandview=articleandid=53:commissioner-general-briefs-mediaandcatid=11:latest-newsandItemid=26.

Government of Ghana. 2010. *Medium-Term Development Policy Framework: Ghana Shared Growth and Development Agenda 2010–2013.Volume 1: Policy Framework*. National Development Planning Commission, Accra.

Health Systems 20/20. 2008. *Another Critique of the Abuja Target*. http://www.healthsystems2020.org/content/blog/detail/2073/.

Heller, P. 2006. "The Prospect of Creating 'Fiscal Space' for the Health Sector." *Health Policy and Planning* 21 (2): 75–79.

IMF (International Monetary Fund). 2011a. *Ghana: 2011 Article IV Consultation*. Washington, DC.

———. 2011b. *Staff Report for the 2011 Article IV Consultation*. Africa Department, Washington, DC.

MOH (Ministry of Health). 2009. *Financial Statements 2009*. Accra.

———. 2010. *Needs Assessment for Implemenation of the WHO Framework Convention on Tobacco Control in Ghana*. Accra.

NHIA (National Health Insurance Authority). 2010. *2009 Annual Report*. Accra.

Owusu-Dabo, E., A. L. McNeil, A. Gilmore, and J. Britton. 2010. "Status of Implementation of Framework Convention on Tobacco Control (FCTC) in Ghana: A Qualitative Study." *BMC Public Health* 10: 1–11.

Saleh, Karima. Forthcoming (2012). *The Health Sector in Ghana: A Comprehensive Assessment.* Washington, DC: World Bank.

Seiter, A. 2011. *Country Status Report: Pharmaceutical Background Paper.* Ministry of Health, Accra, and World Bank, Washington, DC.

Smith, M., and A. Fairbank. 2008. *An Estimate of Potential Costs and Benefits of Adding Family Planning Services to the National Health Insurance Scheme in Ghana and the Impact on the Private Sector.* Banking on Health Project, Accra.

Tandon, A., and C. Cashin. 2010. "Assessing Public Expenditure on Health from a Fiscal Space Perspective." World Bank, Washington, DC.

UNDP (United Nations Development Programme). 2011. *Leveraging Fiscal Space for Human Development in Ghana.* New York.

WHO (World Health Organization). 2005. *Report Card on the WHO Framework Convention on Tobacco Control: Ghana.* Geneva: WHO.

World Bank. 2010. *Poverty Reduction Support Credit Report.* Washington, DC.

———. 2011a. *Republic of Ghana: Joint Review of Public Expenditure and Financial Management.* Africa Region, Country Department West Africa 1, Poverty Reduction and Economic Management 4, Washington, DC.

———. 2011b. *World Development Indicators.* Washington, DC: World Bank. http://data.worldbank.org/data-catalog/world-development-indicators/.

CHAPTER 5

Options for Reforming Health Financing

Ghana is well down the road of transitioning from a supply-side, budget-driven health system to a demand-side financing system, in which money follows patients. Its health reform path is serving as an example for Sub-Saharan Africa—and for low- and middle-income countries throughout the world.

Many aspects of the National Health Insurance Scheme (NHIS) can be considered model good practice. Ghana has made remarkable progress in establishing stable and diverse funding sources for the NHIS, and the new purchasing function is beginning to mature, with the potential to drive fundamental changes in service delivery. Most important, although still in its early days, the NHIS appears to have made a difference for the people of Ghana. Service utilization, which had declined precipitously under the "cash and carry" system, has rebounded. Out-of-pocket spending has declined significantly, there is evidence that the impact of insurance on utilization of health care is highest among the poor, and consumer satisfaction with the system is high.

These achievements notwithstanding, the NHIS faces serious challenges. Current expenditure patterns, driven by the structural features of the system; enrollment inequities; proposed continued expansions; and implementation problems are unsustainable. As a result, the NHIS faces a serious threat of insolvency by 2013 if the trajectory is not altered.

Fundamental reforms are needed in administrative systems, eligibility requirements, the structure of the benefit package, and the way in which providers are paid if the NHIS is to survive and achieve its goals.

This chapter describes options for dealing with the basic design and implementation problems in Ghana's health financing system with a principal focus on the NHIS and in the context of global good practices. Although overall health spending levels and their sustainability are discussed in the context of Ghana's likely future available fiscal space, the emphasis is on the structural and operational reforms to the NHIS needed to ensure its medium- to long-term financial viability in terms of both revenues and expenditures. The financing of basic public health, overall pharmaceutical sector policy, and infrastructure changes are the subjects of other focused reports as well as the Country Status Report (Saleh forthcoming [2012]).

Global Good Practices in Health Financing

All health financing systems are country specific. But global "good practices" can nevertheless help inform policy makers as they design their reform policies.

Good Practices in Health Financing: Lessons from Low- and Middle-Income Countries (Gottret, Schieber, and Waters 2008) identifies 15 "enabling factors" based on 9 "good practice" case studies (Chile, Colombia, Costa Rica, Estonia, the Kyrgyz Republic, Sri Lanka, Thailand, Tunisia, and Vietnam) (table 5.1). These factors are consistent with the factors identified in another World Bank study that also included high-income countries (Gottret and Schieber 2006).

Another World Bank publication, *Governing Mandatory Health Insurance* (Gottret and Savedoff 2008), focuses on governance issues, such as supervisory boards, regulations, and accountability, which have a significant effect on performance and require inclusion within a broader agenda of health reforms (table 5.2). It discusses good practices based on case studies (in Chile, Estonia, and the Netherlands) and other global experience.

The 2010 *World Health Report* (WHO 2010b) and its numerous background papers provide a plethora of empirical and conceptual information on the key issues in establishing universal health insurance coverage. One particularly innovative aspect of the report is an in-depth look at potential efficiency gains, an area much neglected in most studies and one of the most important areas for obtaining additional fiscal space in all countries.

Table 5.3 provides estimates of the potential financial gains from different types of efficiency improvements by country income class. It shows

Table 5.1   Enabling Conditions for Health Reforms

Institutional and societal factors	Policy factors	Implementation factors
• Strong and sustained economic growth • Long-term political stability and sustained political commitment • Strong institutional and policy environment • High levels of population education	• Commitment to equity and solidarity • Health coverage and financing mandates • Financial resources committed to health, including private financing • Consolidation of risk pools • Limits to decentralization • Primary care (first contact care) focus	• Coverage changes accompanied by carefully sequenced health service delivery and provider payment reforms • Good institutional systems and evidence-based decision making • Strong stakeholder support • Use of efficiency gains and co-payments as financing mechanisms • Flexibility and midcourse corrections

Source: Gottret, Schieber, and Waters 2008.

Table 5.2   Governance Factors Related to Mandatory Health Insurance

Dimension	Features
Coherent decision-making structures	• Responsibility for mandatory health insurance objectives corresponds with decision making and capacity in each institution involved in the management of the system. • All mandatory health insurance entities have routine risk assessment and management strategies in place. • The costs of regulating and administering mandatory health insurance institutions are reasonable and appropriate
Stakeholder participation	• Stakeholders have effective representation in the governing bodies of mandatory health insurance.
Transparency and information	• The objectives of mandatory health insurance are formally and clearly defined. • Mandatory health insurance relies on an explicit and appropriately designed institutional and legal framework. • Clear information, disclosure and transparency rules are in place. • Mandatory health insurance entities are subject to minimum requirements with regard to protecting the insured.

(continued next page)

Table 5.2   *(continued)*

Dimension	Features
Supervision and regulation	• Rules on compliance, enforcement, and sanctions for mandatory health insurance supervision are clearly defined. • Financial management rules for mandatory health insurance entities are clearly defined and enforced. • The mandatory health insurance system has structures for ongoing supervision and monitoring in place.
Consistency and stability	• The main qualities of mandatory health insurance system are stable.

Source: Gottret and Savedoff 2008.

savings of 20–40 percent for a comprehensive set of reforms. All of the areas identified—human resources, medicines, hospitals, leakages, and intervention mix—are identified in chapter 3 and the Country Status Report (Saleh forthcoming [2012]) as potential areas for needed reforms in Ghana.

A study of 27 advanced and 23 emerging market countries conducted by the International Monetary Fund (IMF) analyzes the factors responsible for excess growth in health care costs and the effectiveness of measures to contain it (IMF 2010). It provides estimates of the effectiveness of different measures in controlling costs. Of particular interest is the potential effectiveness of extending market mechanisms, improving public sector management, and setting budget caps (box 5.1). Price controls appear to be ineffective.

A 2010 OECD study (*Value for Money in Health Spending*) analyzes the impacts of various policies for limiting public spending on health during periods of constrained budgets. Table 5.4 highlights the range of policies and their likely impacts.

Ghana has many of the enabling conditions for a successful health care reform. But it lacks others, such as limited decentralization and a focus on primary care. Given the unsustainability of the system, the new macro environment, and the mixed performance record of the NHIS, now may be the time for a serious midcourse correction.

Many of the policy tools for controlling health spending are in their development stages in Ghana. Most of the cost containment mechanisms discussed above are absent. Building on the sensible start Ghana has made with respect to diagnosis related groups (DRGs) and primary care capitation, policy makers in the Ministry of Finance and Economic Planning (MOFEP), the NHIS, the Ministry of Health, and the Ghana Health

Table 5.3 Estimated Potential Efficiency Savings in the Health Sector, by Country Income Category and Source

Source of savings	Share of total health spending (percent)		Potential efficiency savings (percent)		Potential efficiency savings (% of total health spending)[a]		Potential efficiency savings per capita ($ billion)[b]		Potential efficiency savings across 1 total population ($ billion)	
	From	To	From	To	From	To	Mean	Range	Mean	Range
Human resources									563	110–851
High-income	55	65	15	25	8	16	492	78–629	499	79–639
Mid-income	45	55	15	25	7	14	14	7–48	61	29–206
Low-income	50	60	15	25	8	15	2	1–5	3	1–6
Medicine									115	24–193
High-income	15	21	10	15	1.5	3	93	14–122	95	14–124
Mid-income	20	30	10	15	2	5	5	2–16	19	9–67
Low-income	25	35	10	15	3	5	1	0–2	1	0–2
Hospitals									287	54–503
High-income	32	42	10	20	3	8	233	30–325	236	31–330
Mid-income	35	45	15	25	5	11	11	5–39	49	23–168
Low-income	27	37	15	25	4	9	1	1–3	2	1–4
Leakages									271	51–468
High-income					3	8	221	28–310	224	29–315
Mid-income					5	10	10	5–35	44	22–150
Low-income					5	10	2	1–3	2	1–4
Intervention-mix									705	141–1,094
High-income					10	20	602	95–774	611	96–786
Mid-income					10	20	21	10–70	89	43–299
Low-income					10	20	3	2–7	4	2–8
Total									1,409	282–2,188
High-income					20	40	1,204	189–1,548	1,223	192–1,573
Mid-income					20	40	42	20–140	178	86–599
Low-income					20	40	7	3–13	8	4–17

Source: WHO 2010b.

a. Derived by multiplying a range of potential efficiency savings (human resources 15–25%; medicine 10–15%; hospitals 10–25%) by share of total health spending in the different country income groups; potential efficiency savings for leakages and intervention mix estimated directly as a percentage of health expenditure per capita (6, 69).

b. Derived by multiplying potential efficiency savings by average health expenditure per capita (interquartile range): 4013 [947–3871] (high-income); 139 [101–351] (middle-income); 22 [15–33] (low-income) (6, 69).

Box 5.1

Macro-, Micro-, and Demand-Side Reforms for Controlling Costs in Advanced Countries

Reforms implemented in advanced countries over the past three decades can be grouped into three categories: macro-level, micro-level, and demand-side reforms.

Macro-level reforms include the following:

- *Budget caps* are the bluntest instrument for restraining resources allocated to the public health sector. They can be expressed as limits on overall health care spending or on subsectors, such as hospitals or pharmaceuticals. Examples include global budgets for hospitals or expenditure ceilings for general practitioners.
- *Supply constraints* regulate the volume of either inputs into or outputs from the health care system. Input controls include limiting admission to physician training colleges, establishing positive lists for drugs, and rationing high-tech capital equipment. Output controls include delisting certain treatments, such as eye tests and dental treatment.
- *Price controls* regulate prices of inputs or outputs. They include wage controls for health care professionals, reference pricing for pharmaceuticals, and price controls on specific treatments.

Micro-level reforms include the following:

- *Public management and coordination reforms* seek to alter the organizational arrangements between different parts of the health care system in order to reduce costs through improved coordination, alignment of responsibility and accountability, better incentive structures, and reduction in overlap or redundancy. Examples of such changes include abolition of managerial levels, decentralization of health care functions, and introduction of gatekeeping arrangements (a system in which a physician who manages a patient's health care services coordinates referrals to secondary and tertiary levels, helping to control health care costs by screening out unnecessary services).
- *Provider reimbursement* is one of the most important factors impacting the micro-level efficiency of health spending. There are many different ways to pay physicians, hospitals, and other providers. Three of the most general methods

(continued next page)

Box 5.1 *(continued)*

include salaries or budgets, case-based payment (such as capitation or diag-
nostic-related groups), and fee-for-service.

• *Market mechanism reforms* seek to improve micro-level efficiency, control
costs, or both by introducing varying degrees of market mechanisms into the
health sector. These reforms operate not so much on the supply side as on the
nexus between supply and demand. Examples include the creation of internal
markets (for example, where primary care physicians purchase services from
hospitals), separating the purchase of health services from provision (thus allowing competition among providers), and promoting patient choice (for example, allowing patients to choose among primary care providers and
hospitals).

Demand-side reforms include policies intended to increase the share of health
care costs borne by patients, often with the objective of avoiding excessive consumption of specific health services. The two most important issues on the
demand side are the level of patient cost-sharing (which can take the form of
lump-sum or percentage copayments) and the tax treatment of private health
insurance.

Source: IMF 2010.

Services are well positioned to carefully assess these mechanisms, which
have differential impacts on access, costs, and quality, and ultimately affect
all aspects of health systems functioning (equity, efficiency, sustainability,
health outcomes, financial protection, and consumer responsiveness). The
hard-learned lessons from the experiences of both high-income and emerging market countries provide an important knowledge base for the design
and implementation of many of the reform options discussed below.

A major precondition for analyzing reform options and transitioning to
full universal coverage is relevant data. It is not possible to run a modern
health system or health insurance scheme without having a modern
health information system in place. Providers need modern financial
management and clinical information systems to capture, collate, and create claims to be sent to payers for payment/reimbursement and quality
assurance as well as to the Ministry of Health and the Ghana Health
Service for disease surveillance, epidemiological monitoring, and health
planning. Much of this infrastructure is still missing in Ghana, as the

Table 5.4 Impacts of Various Policies that Restrain Health Spending

Characteristics, impacts and tradeoffs	Impact on expenditure		Financial protection and access to care	Impact on objectives and trade-offs		
	Strength	Impact lag		Quality of care	Responsiveness	Cost efficiency
A. Macroeconomic policies aimed at expenditure restraint						
A.1 Wage and price controls (labor)	High	Short	None	None/negative	Negative	Positive
A.2 Wage and price controls (medical materials)	High	Short	None	Negative	Negative	Positive
A.3 Controls on volume of inputs (labor)	High	Moderate	None/negative	Negative	Negative	Positive
(capital investment)	High	Short	None/negative	Negative	Negative	Positive
A.4 Controls on volume of other inputs (high tech/drugs)	Moderate	Short	Negative	Negative	Negative	Positive/negative
A.5 Budget caps (sector and global)	High	Short	Negative	Negative	Negative	Positive/negative
A.6 Shift of costs to private sector (increased financing of cost by users)	Moderate	Moderate	Negative	Positive/negative	Positive/negative	Positive
B. Microeconomic policies aimed at increasing efficiency						
B.1 Demand side						
B.1 Disease prevention and health promotion	Low/moderate	Long	Positive	Positive	None	Positive
B.2 Gate-keeping/triaging	Long	Positive	Positive	Positive	Negative	Positive
B.3 Care coordination integrated care/self-care	Moderate	Long	Positive	Positive	Positive/negative	Positive/negative
B.4 Better patient/doctor contact	Low	Moderate	None/positive	Positive	None/positive	Positive/negative

(continued next page)

B.5 Access to primary care doctor out of office hours (to take the pressure off hospital emergency services)	Moderate	Long	Positive	Positive	Positive	Positive
B.2 Supply side						
B.6 Further shift from hospital to ambulatory care	Moderate high	Long	Negative	Positive/negative	Negative	Positive
B.7 Enhancement of the role of health care purchasers	Moderate	Long	Positive/negative	Positive	Positive/negative	Positive
B.8 Improvement of hospital contracting/purchasing/payment systems	Moderate	Long	None	Positive/negative	Positive/negative	Positive
B.9 Increase in managerial independence	Long	Unknown	Positive	Positive/negative	Positive	
B.10 Improvement of payment methods/incentives for hospitals	Moderate	Long	Positive	Positive	Positive/negative	Positive
B.11 Overseeing of technological change and the pricing of medical goods	Moderate/low	Long	Positive/negative	Positive/negative	Positive/negative	Positive
B.12 Increased use of information and communications technology for information transmission	Moderate/low	Long	Positive/negative	Positive	Positive/negative	Positive/negative

Source: OECD 2010.

overall plan for creating a modern information flow has yet to be devised, based on sectorwide standards that all stakeholders follow. For the NHIS, this problem results in serious deficiencies and duplications in membership and registration counts, incomplete claims information and late payments, and errors in financial management.[1]

Several options for reforming the structural basis of the NHIS and improving its operational effectiveness are presented below. Except for the OXFAM proposal to scrap the NHIS in favor of a national health service, these options focus on incremental changes from the current system, not the design of a new one.

Should the National Health Insurance Scheme Be Replaced with a National Health Service?

The most fundamental reform of the health financing system (as proposed in the OXFAM report by Apoya and Marriott 2011) would be to scrap the NHIS and go back to a national health service. Table 5.5

Table 5.5   Arguments for and against Replacing Ghana's National Health Insurance Scheme with a National Health Service

Arguments for (OXFAM's)	Arguments against
• The NHIS is a complete and expensive failure, covering only 18 percent of the population.	• Previous national health service approaches in Ghana resulted in the discredited cash-and-carry system, access and use fell, and the system was inefficient.
• After five years of operation, its administrative processes and health management information system remain extremely deficient.	• The NHIS covers all vulnerable groups and is financed with equitable and efficient earmarked revenues, one of the supposed advantages of a national health service.
• A national health service covers everyone and is more equitable and efficient.	• NHIS financing is largely equitable and efficient, based on general revenues.
• Reliance on a publicly owned and operated delivery system is much more efficient than relying on private sector providers.	• Revenues from the National Health Insurance Levy are earmarked for the poor and other vulnerable groups.
	• Private providers account for about 50 percent of service delivery.
	• Consumer satisfaction with the NHIS is high.
	• The government is committed to expanding the NHIS and making it work more effectively.

Source: Authors.

summarizes the purported advantages and actual disadvantages of this option. It suggests that doing away with the NHIS at this point in its evolution does not make sense.

Both a national health service and a universal mandatory health insurance fund such as the NHIS pool risks and provide financial protection in an insurance sense. Countries need to focus not on generic models but on performing the functions of revenue collection, risk pooling, and purchasing in the most equitable, efficient, and sustainable manner in order to achieve health outcomes, financial protection, and consumer responsiveness.

From a revenue collection prospective, it is argued that general revenues, which are associated with national health service approaches, are a more equitable, efficient, and sustainable revenue source than payroll taxes and other subsidies needed by mandatory health insurance schemes if they are to cover the poor. However, much like a classic national health service model, the NHIS is already funded largely by general revenues, and earmarked national tax subsidies are dedicated for the poor and informal workers, whose premiums are income related. Furthermore, the revenue sources used to finance the NHIS are largely progressive. Given its very low revenue effort and the likely resistance from MOFEP to efforts to further reduce its economic management flexibility by earmarking yet additional revenues to health, seeking additional revenues for further risk pooling from additional general revenue contributions would not appear to be feasible. Instead, obtaining those revenues from individuals able to pay for services (as well as enforcing greater compliance by formal sector firms that are supposed to pay Social Security and National Insurance Trust [SSNIT] taxes) makes good policy sense and could reduce pressure on the government budget. Thus, from the revenue collection side, the NHIS has all the advantages of a national health service approach. It has dealt with the problems often encountered in mandatory health insurance systems of financing the poor and other disadvantaged groups.

In terms of risk pooling, the ultimate goal of the NHIS is to cover the whole population, in the same way a national health service does. Reforming administrative processes, continuing to expand coverage, and providing incentives/penalties for both uninsured informal and formal sector workers to enroll as required by the law will result in risk pooling and coverage for the entire population. From a risk-pooling perspective, there is no difference between a single fund universal health insurance system and a national health service. The key issue under both systems is that for universal coverage to be a reality individuals need to be enrolled and services made available to all beneficiaries. To ensure that this is the case, the government needs to deal with constraints in Ghana's delivery system and the inequitable distribution of resources, whatever financing approach is adopted.

From a purchasing function perspective, the literature does not establish that a government-owned and -operated national health service is always more efficient than a mandatory health insurance system. The issue is the incentives built into the system. Modern payment systems generally require purchaser-provider splits and pay-for-performance provider payment mechanisms, which can be implemented by either the NHIS or a national health service. Indeed, many observers argue that it is easier to install such systems in a mandatory health insurance system than it is to change civil service rules. Moreover, with about half of all NHIS care provided by the private sector, it does not make sense on access and capacity grounds to switch to a fully government-owned system. Ghana's historical experience with the Ministry of Health as a national health service does not bode well for scraping the NHIS and reconstituting the Ministry of Health and its delivery system as Ghana's national insurance entity.

In sum, the general revenue–based financing of the NHIS is largely progressive, equitable, and efficient, and revenues from the National Health Insurance Levy are earmarked for the poor and other vulnerable groups. Private providers account for some 50 percent of service delivery. Consumer satisfaction with the NHIS is high, and the government is committed to expanding the NHIS and make it work effectively.

In view of these factors, OXFAM's recommendation to scrap the NHIS and return to a classic general revenue–funded national health service with no premiums or copayments and a public delivery system does not appear to be a preferred starting or end point on political, analytical policy reform, or sustainability grounds. A better approach is to build on the strengths of the NHIS and to address its weaknesses, most of which would still be present in a national health service. Reform options should focus on reengineering the NHIS and improving its operational effectiveness while concurrent policy reforms in public sector management, public health, the service delivery system, and related areas are undertaken.

Options for Reengineering the National Health Insurance Scheme through Structural Reforms

For the NHIS to function more effectively, reforms should be considered in the following structural features and operational areas: eligibility, the basic benefits package and cost sharing, the contribution base and levels of subsidies, provider payment, pharmaceutical policies, and administration, including the district mutual health insurance schemes (DMHISs) and health management information systems (HMISs). Policy should focus on the following priorities:

1. At least maintaining the share of new revenue (from economic growth or improved revenue collection) allocated to the health sector. Revenue for the NHIS has been stable, growing modestly over time. Except for informal sector enrollees, financing is largely progressive. It should be possible to maintain this trajectory, given the macroeconomic and fiscal projections presented in chapter 4. It would be difficult to argue, however, for dramatically increasing funds to the NHIS given the fragile macroeconomic recovery and fiscal consolidation in Ghana, as well as the current inefficiencies in the NHIS and Ghana's health system more generally. Obtaining additional revenues for spending increases on an inefficient base is not good policy. How money is spent is at least as important as how much money is spent.
2. Ensuring that the full amounts of commitments from all sources are transferred to the NHIF in a timely manner.
3. Optimizing the mobilization of resources within the NHIS through enforced means-tested premiums and possibly strategic copayments in order to add to the revenue base and direct utilization toward more cost-effective services.
4. Assessing the viability of the current benefit package with no cost-sharing.
5. Embarking on strategic purchasing to use provider payment systems and other purchasing tools to contain cost growth, improve the cost-effectiveness of service utilization, and drive efficiencies in the health system.
6. Addressing the severe operational inefficiencies within the NHIS, particularly in processing claims.

Each of these measures is discussed below.

Increasing the Revenues of the National Health Insurance Scheme

Additional revenues can be obtained through a number of mechanisms, including maintaining the NHIS' share of new government revenues and modifying the contribution base and levels of subsidies through a variety of tax and premium-based mechanisms. One must always be conscious of the fact that revenue enhancements other than cost sharing do little to encourage efficient spending. Simply increasing revenues to pay for expansions results in very poor value for money if the base system is inefficient.

Maintaining the share of new government revenue allocated to the NHIS. Prospects for increasing resources for health in Ghana through economic growth and better mobilization of government revenues could be significant, at least over the next five years. Even under the conservative assumption that annual economic growth levels off at a modest 6–7 percent, real government health expenditure could be as much as 45 percent higher in 2015 than in 2009.

As Ghana continues its transition to universal coverage, it is important that the NHIS, and the health sector as a whole, continue to benefit at least proportionally from any government revenue gains. It could be argued that the share should increase slightly, given the moderate share of GDP and the government budget that Ghana currently spends on health as well as the significant expansions of coverage envisioned. Expecting major additional increases in health spending beyond what will be possible from economic growth and improved revenue collection is not realistic, however, given Ghana's fragile macroeconomic recovery and fiscal consolidation.

Modifying the contribution base and the levels of subsidies. There are several ways to increase the contribution base of the NHIS. NHIS contribution rates are not actuarially based. The NHIS is a general revenue–financed program, as the National Health Insurance Levy accounts for 61 percent of program revenues and more than 75 percent of revenues if investment income (which will be gone by 2013) and donor contributions (which may disappear given Ghana's newfound lower-middle-income country status) are excluded. Adding in the other national revenue source, the SSNIT, brings the share of revenues from national taxes to 77 percent. Excluding investment income and donor support means that the value added tax (VAT) and SSNIT account for 95 percent of program revenues.

Increasing earmarked taxes. Options frequently considered for increasing revenues include the following:

- increasing the VAT earmark
- increasing the 2.5 percentage point SSNIT contribution dedicated to health from the 18.5 percent SSNIT tax, by increasing the tax rate or reallocating a larger share of the tax to health

- earmarking revenues from the current or increased cigarette and alcohol excise taxes to health.

Table 5.6 summarizes the pros and cons of increasing the VAT and SSNIT earmarks.

Increasing the VAT or SSNIT earmarks, either through an increase in rates or by reallocating a larger percentage to the health sector, is likely to inhibit fiscal management by reducing the flexibility of the government to reallocate funds across sectors. Increasing the SSNIT rate and earmarking the additional revenues to health is likely to have adverse effects on labor markets and employment, possibly increasing informality. Reallocating a larger percentage of SSNIT revenues is highly unlikely given the weak financial position of the Social Security Pension Fund. Furthermore, current revenues earmarked to health from the VAT and SSNIT account for some 5 percent of total government tax revenues just for NHIS. It is not likely that the government would be willing to earmark additional revenues from these sources, further reducing its fiscal management flexibility. From a policy perspective, the government may not

Table 5.6   Arguments for and against Increasing the Value Added Tax (VAT) and Social Security and National Insurance Trust (SSNIT) Earmarks to Fund Ghana's National Health Insurance Scheme

Arguments for	Arguments against
• The VAT accounted for 61 percent of 2009 NHIS revenues; the SSNIT accounted for 16 percent. Increasing either tax through higher rates (or in the case of SSNIT, reallocating more of it to health) could solve the sustainability problem of the NHIS. • As the VAT is very broad based, relatively efficient, and equitable, it is an excellent candidate for revenue enhancement.	• Revenue enhancements do little to deal with underlying inefficiencies in the NHIS and the health system more generally. • Pouring large volumes of new funds into an inefficient base system is not a recommended policy option. • As the current VAT and SSNIT earmarks account for some 5 percent of overall government tax revenues, the Ministry of Finance and Economic Planning is likely to strongly resist further earmarking, which reduces its macroeconomic management flexibility. • Increases in the SSNIT would likely reduce employment and encourage informality. • Reallocation of the pension portion of the SSNIT to health is unlikely, as the pension system is also in financial crisis.

Source: Authors.

want to increase the already high level of cross-subsidization from the SSNIT NHIS category of eligibles to all other NHIS eligibility groups. On revenue generation (and possibly equity) grounds, a broader-based tax might make more sense.

Another option would be to impose additional excise taxes on alcohol and tobacco ("sin taxes"). Table 5.7 summarizes the pros and cons doing so.

Both cigarette and alcohol consumption are low in Ghana, and revenues from these excise taxes currently account for only some 1–2 percent of total tax revenues. Tobacco products are taxed at a rate of only about 29 percent—far lower than the average rate in Africa of 40 percent or the WHO-recommended rate of 70 percent (WHO 2010a). Alcohol taxes and consumption are also low in Ghana, although as in the case of cigarettes there is a complex tiered rate structure (WHO 2009, 2011).

Given the relatively small sizes of the markets, low tax rates, and complex tiered rate structures, it would appear to be feasible to double revenues from these taxes, resulting in additional tax revenues of about GH¢100 million or about one-third of NHIS income if all the increased revenues were earmarked to the NHIS (Stenberg and others 2010). These

Table 5.7   Arguments for and against Increasing Sin Taxes Earmarked to Fund Ghana's National Health Insurance Scheme

Arguments for	Arguments against
• Sin taxes, such as excise taxes on alcohol and tobacco, are a popular form of revenue generation, on the grounds of both reducing externalities and raising revenue, as demand for these products is inelastic. Both cigarette and alcohol consumption are low in Ghana, and revenues from these excise taxes currently account for only 1–2 percent of total tax revenues. However, it has been estimated that simplifying the rate structures and increasing tax rates could result in some GH¢100–GH¢150 million in additional revenues, on the order of one-third of current NHIS income. In addition, sin taxes would reduce future health care costs and NHIS liabilities by discouraging consumption of products that lead to higher health risks and road accidents.	• Although sin tax increases are feasible and justifiable, it is unlikely that the Ministry of Finance and Economic Planning will agree to further earmarking of revenues to NHIS. • Although cigarette and alcohol taxes would reduce NHIS spending over the medium term, thanks to reductions in the burden of disease, they do little to deal with the base inefficiencies in NHIS structural and operational features and the Ghana health system.

Source: Authors.

tax hikes would also reduce future health care costs and NHIS liabilities by discouraging consumption of products that lead to greater health risks and road accidents. Although there is a vast literature justifying such taxes and the situation in Ghana is favorable for increasing rates (for example, the market is probably too small and prices too low to encourage major smuggling operations), earmarking these additional revenues to health faces many of the same fiscal management flexibility issues as further earmarks of the VAT and SSNIT. A tax increase on these products is justifiable, and such additional revenues could be a viable source of revenues for NHIS, if the government is willing to earmark these funds.

Generating additional premium income. Premium income can be increased in a number of ways, including by requiring people in the top two wealth quintiles who fall into one of the groups that is currently exempt from NHIS premiums to pay premiums and by levying a one-time premium on enrollees.

Charging premiums for currently exempt enrollees who are able to pay is a potentially equitable and significant way to increase premium income. About 65 percent of enrollees in the NHIS belong to groups that are exempt from premium fees. Some groups (for example, pregnant women and the poor) are also exempt from paying the registration fee. Table 5.8 summarizes the pros and cons of removing the exemption status for members of these groups who fall in the top two wealth quintiles.

Table 5.8   Arguments for and against Charging Premiums for Ghana's National Health Insurance Scheme to Currently Exempt Enrollees Able to Pay

Arguments for	Arguments against
• Of the approximately two-thirds of NHIS members who are exempt from premium payments, more than 30 percent are in the top two wealth quintiles of the population and could afford to pay premiums. Charging them the minimal informal sector worker premium of GH¢8 would have generated additional revenues to the NHIS of about GH¢25 million, or some 7 percent of its 2008 income. It would also result in improved equity and better targeting of the NHIL toward the poor.	• Charging such premiums would be politically unpopular. • These groups might drop their coverage and refuse to enroll. • It's not clear that the government or the NHIS have effective tools for undertaking such targeting.

Source: Authors.

The vast scale of exemptions places a heavy financing burden on the National Health Insurance Levy and necessitates large cross-subsidies from nonsubsidized paying groups, such as formal sector workers. Requiring some level of payment from members of exempt groups that are able to pay makes sense on both sustainability and equity grounds. Very rough estimates from the 2008 Monitoring and Evaluation Survey indicate that 46 percent of children and elderly people—who account for about 80 percent of all NHIS exemptions—are in the top two wealth quintiles of the population.[2] Charging them the minimal informal worker premium of GH¢8 would have resulted in additional revenues to the NHIS of GH¢25 million in 2008—some 7 percent of its revenue.

A perhaps slightly more politically acceptable version of this proposal would be to charge exempt individuals from the upper income quintiles a higher registration fee rather than dropping their exemption from premiums. The key operational issue is whether the NHIS has or could put in place the systems needed to be conduct means testing, which is problematic in most countries, including advanced economies.[3] The NHIS would also need to monitor the impact of this policy to ensure that people did not drop out of the NHIS once their exemption was removed.

Another policy option for increasing revenues that is very much on the government's policy agenda is establishment of a one-time premium for lifetime enrollment. This policy has been widely discussed and debated in Ghana. What has been missing is a clear definition of exactly what is meant by a one-time premium.[4] For purposes of this analysis, the one-time premium is interpreted to be a one-time payment for lifetime NHIS coverage. Table 5.9 summarizes the pros and cons of this proposal.

Although all the details for the proposal have not been specified, it is likely that it would apply only to nonexempt groups; SSNIT contributors would also probably not be affected, as they would continue to contribute through the payroll tax. Thus, the payment would fall largely on informal workers and any others (spouses of SSNIT contributors) who are required to pay premiums. In its purest form, the proposal establishes a lifetime "health annuity" with the NHIS for the policyholder. For a one-time premium payment, the individual receives lifetime coverage for the NHIS basic benefits package.

The proposal would simplify enrollment, ensure continuous lifetime coverage, bring in additional revenues in the short run, and allow the NHIS to become a vested system (that is, if actuarially based, its reserves would be adequate to pay for the future liabilities of its premium-paying

Table 5.9   Arguments for and against Charging a One-Time Premium for Lifetime Enrollment in Ghana's National Health Insurance Scheme

Arguments for	Arguments against
• A one-time premium simplifies enrollment, reduces administrative costs, and ensures lifetime continuous coverage. • A one-time premium brings in additional NHIS revenues in the short run. • A one-time premium potentially allows the NHIS to become a "vested" sustainable system (that is, if actuarially based, its reserves would be adequate to pay the future liabilities of its premium-paying enrollees) as opposed to its current status as a pay-as-you-go system (requiring annual appropriated or earmarked revenues).	• Most enrollees would not be able to afford premiums of GH¢665– GH¢1,200 (based on an actuarially sound premium for a young person enrolling in the NHIS), causing them to drop coverage. • The one-time premium violates the insurance element of risk pooling over the individual's life cycle by forcing payment for a lifetime of health liabilities up front instead of spacing/smoothing payments and using them over the enrollee's life cycle, as in the case of medical savings accounts. • Only 29 percent of NHIS enrollees pay premiums (which account for only 3.8 percent of NHIS revenues). If individuals do not enroll because they cannot afford the premium, both revenue generation and coverage would decline. • Heavily subsidizing the premium to encourage enrollment would create a major future contingent liability on the NHIS, necessitating financing from other sources and further compromising sustainability.

Source: Authors.

enrollees) as opposed to its current status as a pay-as-you-go system (requiring annual appropriated or earmarked revenues). In terms of affordability, revenue-raising capacity, and sustainability, however, the lifetime premium faces several serious practical and conceptual challenges.

First, an actuarially sound premium for a young person enrolling in the NHIS should reflect his or her discounted expected future lifetime NHIS costs (that is, 52 years of payments for an 18-year-old informal worker). A recent actuarial report using three estimated premium level scenarios finds that the premium would have to be on the order of GH¢665–GH¢1,200 (Hendriks 2010). Even if the premium were subsidized by as much as 50 percent, few Ghanaians could afford them—and the government could not easily afford the subsidies. No major health insurance system funds its operations this way; health annuities are rare.[5] Unless an individual has substantial assets, a lifetime health "insurance" annuity would not be affordable unless the individual could spread the payments over his or life cycle (as is the case in medical savings accounts). In this way, individuals pool their health risks and payments over the life cycle, building up equity when they are young and have low risks and rising income and drawing down on their equity later in life, when they have higher health risks and lower income.

As few people could afford to pay the premium, many would simply not enroll. Under the current system, only about 29 percent of NHIS enrollees pay premiums (which account for just 3.8 percent of NHIS revenues). If individuals do not enroll because they cannot afford the premiums, both revenue generation and coverage would decline. Worse still, if, as under the present situation, the premium is heavily subsidized to encourage enrollment, there would be a major future contingent liability on the NHIS, necessitating financing from other sources.

The other major problem with the lifetime premium is that it is not sustainable, for two reasons. First, as just mentioned, if subsidized, it would create a large, difficult to predict future liability on the NHIS, threatening its financial sustainability. If this liability could not be covered by earmarked sources or investment earnings, budgetary allocations would be needed to cover it. Second, if everyone enrolled and current exemption levels were maintained, there would be relatively few additional new enrollees each subsequent year, resulting in very limited future revenues.

Thus, despite the appeal of a single lifetime premium in terms of encouraging enrollment, reducing administrative costs, ensuring continuity of coverage, and generating short-run revenues, the concept falls short on basic insurance/risk-pooling, affordability, revenue-raising, and sustainability grounds. Moreover, as it would likely require significant subsidization, it would also create large future contingent cost liabilities. Although premium contributions have the important advantage of spreading risks over the entire population (as opposed to cost sharing, which taxes only people who use services), a lifetime premium is simply not a feasible mechanism. It potentially creates more problems than it solves. Other, more effective mechanisms can accomplish its purported goals.

Summary. All of these options need to be considered in the context of Ghana's institutional realities. Although additional revenues will accrue to the NHIS from its earmarked funding sources as the economy grows, they will not be sufficient to sustain the NHIS once its reserves are depleted in 2013.

Ghana's low revenue effort suggests that tax reforms hold the prospect of increasing the yields of the various tax bases, including the VAT. Given the current heavy earmarking of funds to the NHIS though the National Health Insurance Levy, however—with the resultant rigidities created for macroeconomic management—it is questionable whether the government would consider earmarking additional VAT revenues to the NHIS. Given the weak financial situation of the social security pension fund, additional allocations from the SSNIT are also unlikely. Obtaining increased revenues from sin taxes would appear to be a viable option, but the overall revenue potential is low, given low rates of alcohol and tobacco use, and the earmarking question remains. Making higher-income exempt groups contribute appears to be a sensible option on equity and revenue-generation grounds, but policy makers need to explore its operational feasibility, as well as both the enrollment and political consequences. The lifetime premium, while having certain advantages, is not likely to achieve its desired goals.

Reducing NHIS Expenditure

Expenditures can be reduced though a variety of measures including changes in eligibility criteria and the benefits package, provider payment reforms, pharmaceutical reforms, and administrative improvements. More generally, whether Ghana can afford universal coverage depends on a large number of interrelated factors pertaining to the design of the program and the country's overall fiscal situation. The government is committed to universal coverage. The question is whether it can

- afford a basic benefits package that covers 95 percent of the burden of disease
- maintain a policy of no cost sharing and the consequent loss of revenues, as well as the moral hazard/increased costs such a policy engenders
- operate the program efficiently without effective gatekeepers or referral systems
- use provider payment mechanisms that are not performance-based
- exempt from contributions large numbers of individuals who can afford to pay
- operate without fully automating its HMIS and improving quality assurance, fraud detection, financial systems, and provider certification systems

- continue to use financing arrangements that are not actuarially sound
- reinsure the DMHISs on an open-ended basis.

Changing the eligibility criteria. Everyone in Ghana except members of the military and the police is supposed to enroll in the NHIS. Can Ghana afford universal coverage? Do the eligibility categories make sense? How is universal enrollment (as opposed to eligibility) ensured?

If Ghana wants to provide universal coverage, it will need to carefully design all elements of the program to make the program equitable, efficient, affordable, and sustainable while producing the desired results in terms of access, health outcomes, and financial protection. Alternatively, if resources are too tight, it could consider focusing the program only on the poor and near poor and reducing subsidies to better-off groups, which could buy private insurance or pay actuarially-based premiums for NHIS coverage.

A second issue concerning eligibility is the definition and overlaps of the eligibility groups themselves. Many have argued that the definition of indigent is much too narrow and should be revised. Others question whether enrollment should be family-based rather than individual-based. Does it make sense, for example, for a spouse of someone who pays the SSNIT tax to pay the informal worker premium? Dealing with these issues could improve enrollment, simplify administration, and increase equity.

A third issue pertains to the need to develop mechanisms that ensure that everyone who is eligible for coverage either voluntarily enrolls or is automatically enrolled. Classic solutions involve incentivizing enrollment, through the following mechanisms:

- using private and social marketing methods
- designing an attractive benefits package at affordable prices, and offering different benefit packages for different enrollee groups
- marketing benefits to larger groups (through cooperatives, for example)
- marketing insurance alongside complementary products, such as microcredit (World Bank 2011).

Absent some fundamental changes, adverse selection and low enrollments will continue. Many informal workers do not enroll in the NHIS, because they do not understand the value of insurance. The NHIS needs to do a better job of setting premiums and conducting means testing, given the regressive nature of premiums. Formal sector employers and employees may try to evade the 18.5 percent SSNIT (13 percent falls on the employer and 5.5 percent on the employee, of which 2.5 percentage points of the total contributions are earmarked for health), keeping what would otherwise be income to the government. This phenomenon is well documented in Latin America, where high social security taxes have led to increased labor force informality despite significant economic growth (Baeza and Packard 2006).

Getting formal sector employers to enroll their employees is a matter of tax compliance; enrolling informal workers is more difficult. Getting such workers to enroll voluntarily is a major problem in all countries, and adverse selection continues to be a problem even when premiums are highly subsidized. After unsuccessfully attempting to encourage voluntary enrollments, Thailand simply covered all informal workers, financing them through general revenues rather than premiums, as many were near the poverty line. Given the small share of revenue informal workers currently account for (3.8 percent) and the likelihood that many of the remaining uninsured are probably at or near the poverty line, Ghana should consider a similar solution if the needed financing could be obtained through other revenue enhancements or efficiency improvements. Some or perhaps all of the costs could be offset by more timely diagnosis and treatment.

Modifying the basic benefits package. The basic benefit package covers 95 percent of the burden of disease and includes no cost sharing. Like all health insurance funds, the NHIS faces difficulties coordinating its basic benefits package with vertical public health services financed and provided by the Ministry of Health.

The extensiveness of the basic benefits package could augur a future cost explosion as supply-side constraints are relaxed and the health transition runs its course. All countries ration health services through supply-side constraints, some deliberately (as in the former Soviet Union), others because they lack the human resources to scale up their health systems or simply cannot afford to do so.

For universal coverage to become a reality, program beneficiaries must have access to services. To provide those services effectively, the NHIS must pay no less than it costs to provide such services efficiently. Thus, the government must decide which services will be covered and accessible (that is, supply-side expansions) and develop mechanisms to encourage efficient production and consumption.

Making these decisions often involves tradeoff between cost-effectiveness and financial protection. Can the NHIS encourage efficient consumption in the absence of cost sharing and effective gatekeeper and referral systems? In addition to preventing moral hazard, cost sharing is an additional revenue source, which can be equitable if the poor are exempted. Better harmonization with the Ministry of Health regarding the basic benefits package and vertical public health programs is essential, particularly given Ghana's relatively poor health outcome performance. A study for the U.S. Agency for Development (USAID) shows large potential savings from better coordination of family planning services (Smith and Fairbank 2008). A World Bank marginal budgeting for bottlenecks (MBB) study reinforced the need for better coordination (El Idrissi 2007).

Streamlining provider payment. Various provider payment and cost containment reforms can lead to significant savings by improving efficiency. The current provider payment system is a mélange of supply-side subsidies to public providers from the Ministry of Health in the form of wage and other operating subsidies and NHIS reimbursements based on fee schedules and the Ghana Diagnosis Related Group (G-DRG) system. Fee schedules for private providers are adjusted upward to reflect the absence of public subsidies. These payment systems are a good start in the movement toward strategic purchasing.

Providers are now accustomed to output-oriented payment systems rather than fixed budgets. The uncapped fee-for-service approach does not help the NHIS achieve efficiency, cost-effectiveness of service utilization, cost containment, quality improvement, or equity. Insurance systems in many countries are moving away from traditional fee-for-service payment models toward some combination of bundled payment, blended payment, managed care, and pay-for-performance systems (Rosenthal 2008; Mechanic and Altman 2009). Significant efficiency gains could be achieved by adopting state-of-the-art pay-for-performance systems, which rely on gatekeepers and enforced referral systems.

The NHIS is piloting a primary care capitation model in Ashanti region, as well as other forms of results-based financing. Movement toward capitation may be the first step toward shifting reimbursement toward primary care and rewarding successful prevention efforts, as providers retain any surplus they generate from keeping their population healthy. The capitation pilot will also test the inclusion of basic primary care medicines in the capitated rate to begin to limit the unchecked pharmaceutical expenditures of the NHIS. The pilot represents a first step toward better integrating service delivery, because it encourages providers to form groups to deliver the full range of services in the primary care package funded under capitation. These efforts are in their design stages and will require time to test and evaluate.

All payment systems have upsides and downsides. Ghana's challenge is to employ the appropriate mix of methods to maximize access, macro and micro efficiency, and quality. Although it is likely that reforms will yield savings over the medium to long term, upfront investments will be needed now. Payment reforms are a less painful way to finance the system than eligibility changes, benefit cuts, or larger contributions from individuals. If properly designed, they can simultaneously help the NHIS meet efficiency, access, and quality goals.

Reforming pharmaceutical policies. The NHIS is a key component of pharmaceutical sector policy (the pharmaceutical sector is analyzed in detail in a separate background report [Seiter 2011]). Pharmaceuticals account for an estimated 40–50 percent of NHIS spending.

NHIS coverage of pharmaceuticals has made medicines affordable to enrollees and increased their financial protection, as drugs are one of the biggest components of out-of-pocket spending. Therefore, policy changes in this area have critical implications for the sustainability of the NHIS as well as its performance in terms of health outcomes and financial protection.

The NHIS suffers from several pharmaceutical-related problems, including inappropriate charging for medicines, fraud, overprescribing, and irrational use and prescribing patterns. Better information and claims management systems, improved (risk-based) provider payment systems, copayments, review of the NHIS drug list for medical appropriateness, and changes to NHIS policy on provider and consumer information are recommended. Reimbursement of expenses for generic medicines could be reduced if providers could agree on a pooled purchasing mechanism with framework contracts with suppliers. Such a strategy could also be used to ensure consistent quality of medicines reimbursed by the NHIS. Fraudulent claims account for an estimated 5 percent of NHIS medicine claims (that is, almost 2.5 percent of NHIS spending); overprescribing/abuse accounts for about another 20 percent of medicine expenditures (that is, almost 10 percent of NHIS spending). Reforms in this area could thus lead to significant expenditure reductions and improved health outcomes.

Implementing administrative reform. Administrative changes are essential if the NHIS is to function efficiently as a modern insurer covering more than 20 million people and provide accurate information on beneficiaries, providers, and services. Modernizing and automating the HMIS nationally, within the Ministry of Health, in the NHIS, and for providers is critical. Now that the DMHISs are, for all practical purposes, becoming branches of the NHIS, it may be time to formally convert them into such and consolidate claims payment and enrollment functions, in order to maximize economies of scale and scope. Doing so may require fundamental legal and regulatory changes; some short-term transition cost may have to be incurred in order to achieve savings over the longer term.

Administrative issues are often tedious and deal with operational, as opposed to the more interesting structural, issues. If the NHIS wants to expand coverage, become an "active purchaser," and effectively regulate the health sector, it must upgrade its information systems and deal with previously identified nuts and bolts administrative issues. These issues include the following:

- difficulty identifying poor people
- weak portability
- unreliable eligibility authentication at provider site
- weak control systems, which potential for fraud
- weak enforcement of gatekeeper (referral) system
- high cost of administrative inefficiencies
- gaps in human capacity
- artificial indebtedness
- fragmented claims processing
- misapplication of approved tariffs
- prescribing and dispensing of unapproved medicines
- inefficient medical supply chain system, leading to the high cost of medicines on the NHIS medicines list
- inability to effectively monitor service utilization and cost
- inability to gather timely data on disease patterns, hampering decision making
- manual processing of claims, leading to delayed claims payment
- potential for fraud by enrollees, DMHISs, and providers (Nyonator 2010a, 2010b, 2010c; Seddoh, Adjei, and Nazzar 2011).

Next Steps

The NHIS has a broad agenda. It must deal with both operational issues and structural reforms. It must improve its operational processes and information system. It must establish a modern HMIS and develop much better data for decision making. Its mounting financial deficit is structural in nature; dealing with it is a matter of urgency.

Its top priority is the need to collect up-to-date actuarial information about NHIS enrollment, solvency, and the cost of various reform options. As these reform options span almost the full spectrum of structural composition and operational areas (eligibility criteria, the basic benefits package, contribution arrangements, provider payment, pharmaceuticals, and so forth), an extensive range of data and analyses will be needed—on the costs of alternative basic benefits packages, the implications of charging premiums to some members of exempt groups, the impacts of various cost-sharing options on revenue and utilization, reform of provider payment systems, and so forth.

In parallel, NHIS operational capabilities need to be upgraded. Throughout the process, policymakers must not lose sight of what the NHIS is trying to accomplish: improve health outcomes and provide significantly better financial protection in an equitable, efficient, and sustainable manner. Table 5.10 summarizes the reform areas and some of the options discussed above.

NHIS reforms do not take place in a vacuum; they must be integrated into Ghana's overall health reform agenda. Structural and operational changes that are essential to ensure the viability and sustainability of the NHIS will take time. And major reforms will require upfront investments, many outside the NHIS.

The government should make a commitment to the investment and structural changes needed in the delivery system. High priorities could include rationalization of direct payments from the NHIS to the Ministry of Health and the Ghana Health Service; paying more attention to public health issues; and improving coordination among vertical public health programs, programs of other health-related sectors, and the NHIS basic benefits package. Similar efforts by the Ministry of Health and the Ghana Health Service to expand delivery system capacity are critical, given concerns about physical and human infrastructure access, maldistribution of resources, and quality.

Beyond political willingness, commitment, and ability, a sine qua non for success is the establishment of an accountable, culturally and politically sensitive, and effective reform process that holistically deals with the wide set of issues underlying any major health reform effort. Health financing cannot be viewed in isolation from other health system issues. Taking a holistic view is particularly important given many of the identified weaknesses in the management, organization, and incentives of the entire health care delivery system, including public health programs. If Ghana is to achieve universal coverage, NHIS enrollees must have "effective access"

Table 5.10   Options for Reforming Ghana's National Health Insurance Scheme

Issue	Option
Eligibility for premium subsidies and enrollment changes	• Focus on the poor • Change the eligibility unit from the individual to the household • Create incentives to encourage enrollment
Basic benefits package	• Review extensiveness • Consider cost sharing for the nonpoor • Coordinate with vertical public health programs
Revenues	• Increase the VAT earmark • Increase the SSNIT contribution • Impose sin taxes • Means test exempt groups • Levy a one-time premium on enrollees
Provider payment	• Implement payment systems that encourage efficiency, quality, cost-effective service utilization, and better coordination across the continuum of care; options include the appropriate mix of capitation, other bundled payment systems, blended payment systems, various managed care approaches, and modern pay-for-performance systems
Pharmaceuticals	• Establish more rational reimbursement methods, including capitation for basic primary care medicines, bundling by G-DRGs, reference pricing, or other modern reimbursement methods • Improve information systems and introduce incentives for the rational use of medicines • Update the drug list based on medical appropriateness criteria • Reduce expenditure for generic medicines through pooled procurement • Consider appropriate copayments • Provide consumer and provider education
Administrative reforms	• Provide data for decision making • Improve the HMIS • Centralize control • Adopt other operational reforms
Other	• Strengthen public health • Invest in physical and human infrastructure • Improve governance

Source: Authors.

to services when they need them, and services must be both physically and financially accessible in addition to being medically appropriate and effective. This process must be informed by data and analysis.

Election years are challenging times for all countries. However, now would be an ideal time to get the reform process established and moving, so that the needed analyses can be conducted and policy options costed. Acting now would allow for difficult political decisions to be made right after the December 2012 election, in sufficient time to avoid the bankruptcy of the NHIS in 2013.

Notes

1. For the purposes of estimating rough orders of magnitude, this study used information from the NHIS annual report. These data should not be used for precise point estimates (see Hendriks 2010).

2. Under current arrangements, children 18 and under are covered if both parents are NHIS members. Legislation is pending to drop the parent enrolment requirement.

3. Given the regressivity of the premiums for informal workers, it is important for the NHIS to do a much better job enforcing its means testing. It is not surprising that the premium is regressive, as most enrollees pay near the minimum. Of course, one needs to consider the level of subsidy on the benefit side as well. Further analysis is required to obtain a complete picture of the net benefit incidence.

4. See Saleh (forthcoming [2012]) and Seddoh, Adjei, and Nazzar (2011) for discussions of both the ambiguity problem and the politics.

5. Individuals in the United States can sign over their assets to a nursing home in exchange for a guarantee of future lifetime care.

References

Apoya, P., and A. Marriott. 2011. *Achieving a Shared Goal: Free Universal Health Care in Ghana.* Alliance for Reproductive Health Rights, Essential Services Platform of Ghana, Integrated Social Development Centre and Oxfam International, United Kingdom.

Baeza, C., and T. Packard. 2006. *Beyond Survival, Protecting Households from Health Shocks in Latin America.* World Bank, Washington, DC, and Stanford University, Stanford, CA.

El Idrissi, M. 2007. *Summary of Bottleneck Analysis used for the MBB (Mainly MDG 4, 5 and 6), 2007 and Connection with the Health System.* Washington, DC, World Bank.

Gottret, P., and W. Savedoff. 2008. *Governing Mandatory Health Insurance.* World Bank, Washington, DC.

Gottret, P., and G. Schieber. 2006. *Health Financing Revisited.* World Bank, Washington, DC.

Gottret, P., G. Schieber, and H. Waters. 2008. *Good Practices in Health Financing: Lessons from Low- and Middle-Income Countries.* World Bank, Washington, D.C.

Hendriks, R. 2010. *National Health Insurance Ghana.* World Bank, Washington, DC, and Ghana Ministry of Health, Accra.

IMF (International Monetary Fund). 2010. *Macro-Fiscal Implications of Health Care Reform in Advanced and Emerging Economies.* Fiscal Affairs Department, Washington, DC.

Mechanic, R., and S. Altman. 2009. "Payment Reform Options: Episode Payment Is a Good Place to Start." *Health Affairs* 28 (2): w262–271.

Nyonator, F. 2010a. *District Mutual Health Insurance Scheme Operations in Ghana: Key Operational Components, Quality Assurance and Challenges, PowerPoint Presentation.* World Bank Institute, Washington, DC:

———. 2010b. "Establishment and Governance of the National Health Insurance Scheme (NHIS) Based on District Mutual Health Insurance Schemes." PowerPoint Presentation, World Bank Institute, Washington, DC.

———. 2010c. *Ghana Case Study.* World Bank Institute Health Reform Flagship Course, Washington, DC.

OECD (Organization for Economic Co-operation and Development). 2010. *Value for Money in Health Spending.* Paris: OECD.

Rosenthal, M. 2008. "Beyond Pay for Performance: Emerging Models of Provider Payment Reform." *New England Journal of Medicine* 359 (12): 1197–1200.

Saleh, Karima. Forthcoming (2012). *The Health Sector in Ghana: A Comprehensive Assessment.* Washington, DC: World Bank.

Seddoh, A., S. Adjei, and A. Nazzar. 2011. *Ghana's National Health Insurance Scheme.* Rockefeller Foundation, New York.

Seiter, A. 2011. "Country Status Report: Pharmaceutical Background Paper." Ministry of Health, Accra, and World Bank, Washington, DC.

Smith, M., and A. Fairbank. 2008. *An Estimate of Potential Costs and Benefits of Adding Family Planning Services to the National Health Insurance Scheme in Ghana and the Impact on the Private Sector.* Banking on Health Project, Accra.

Stenberg, K. R. Elovainio, D. Chisholm, D. Fuhr, A.-M., Perucic, D. Rekve, and A. Yurekli. 2010. *Responding to the Challenge of Resource Mobilization: Mechanisms for Raising Additional Domestic Resources for Health.* Background Paper 13, World Health Report 2010, World Health Organization, Geneva.

WHO (World Health Organization). 2009. *Report on the Global Tobacco Epidemic 2009: Implementing Smoke-Free Environments.* Geneva.

———. 2010a. *Ghana Report Card on the WHO Framework Convention on Tobacco Control.* Geneva.

———. 2010b. *World Health Report.* Geneva: WHO.

———. 2011. *Global Status Report on Alcohol and Health.* Geneva: WHO.

World Bank. 2011. *Philippines Health Sector Review.* Washington, DC and Manila.